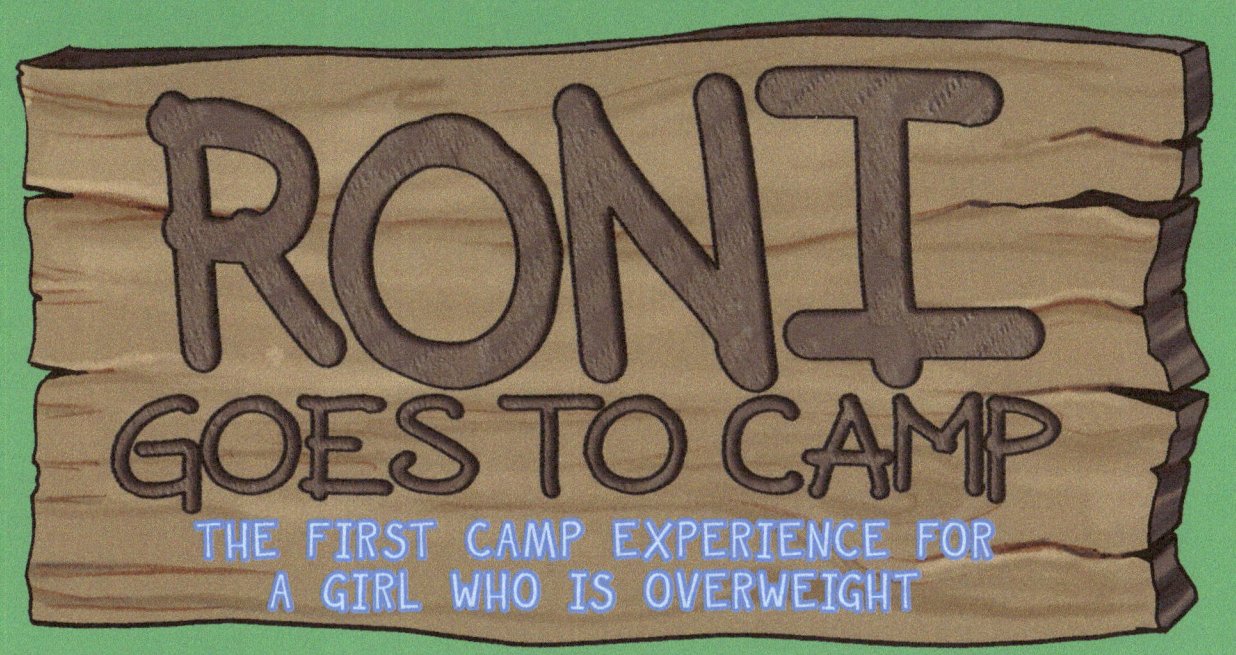

Written By:
Roni Roth Beshears, EdD, RDN
Registered Dietitian Nutritionist

Illustrated By:
Rob Peters

Copyright @ 2015 Nutrition Associates, LLC

All rights reserved. No part of this book may be reproduced, transmitted, or stored in an information retrieval system in any form or by any means, graphic, electronic, or mechanical, including photography, taping, and recording, without prior written permission from the author.

First U.S. edition 2015 (Chubby Roni Goes to Camp)
Second U.S. edition 2016 (Roni Goes To Camp)
First Hardcover edition 2019 (Roni Goes To Camp)

ISBN-13: 978-0-578-57051-8

Illustrations were done by Rob Peters in pen, ink, and 6B pencil on Bristol paper and digitally painted in Photoshop.

All matters regarding weight management and health require medical supervision. The author is not engaged in rendering professional advice or services to children and their families or caregivers. The ideas, procedures, and suggestions contained in this book are not intended as substitutes for consulting with your medical-care provider. All matters regarding summer camps and their policies and practices should be directed to appropriate camp personnel and the American Camp Association. The author shall not be liable or responsible for any loss or damage allegedly arising from information or suggestions in this book. The author does not assume any responsibility for errors or for changes that occur after publication. The author does not have any control over and does not assume any responsibility for author or third-party websites or their content.

To contact Dr. Roni Roth Beshears and to schedule a book and program presentation, please email her at roni.nutritionassociates@gmail.com.

Roni Goes to Camp is the second illustrated children's book in a series of fictionalized true stories on weight management and lifestyle choices for young children who are overweight. The story suggests how the summer camp experience can offer children who are overweight, especially young girls, valuable lessons in self-awareness and self-management, with the help of supportive staff and counselors. It also shows how camp can provide an opportunity for children to learn and develop positive health and lifestyle behaviors to last a lifetime.

The first book in this series, *Roni Takes Action*, is about a young girl who is overweight and teased by schoolmates and embarrassed by her unsatisfactory school physical fitness report. With the help of a dietitian, Roni and her family take action to improve their diet and health. The story offers simple and practical changes to guide children who are overweight to achieve a balanced and healthy lifestyle with family support.

The *Roni Children's Book Series* is an educational and engaging teaching tool for school-age children who are overweight and their families. Roni is a strong and confident young girl who wants to empower children to develop a positive self-image and embrace a healthy lifestyle.

Places for book distribution are homes, libraries, schools, community centers, and medical practices. The series supports the establishment of nonthreatening and wholesome environments to help children who are overweight grow, learn, and accomplish their dreams.

Thanks to:
Rob Peters for creating the book illustrations.
Carol Barkin for editorial consultation and suggestions.
Family, friends, and professional colleagues for reviewing the manuscript.

For Dad:
Who loved summer camp
— RRB

Going to sleep-away camp was scary for me. I had never spent time away from home without my parents.

"I loved camp when I was your age," Dad said to me. "Roni, you'll see—you'll learn to play new sports and make lots of friends. Don't worry, you'll have a great time!"

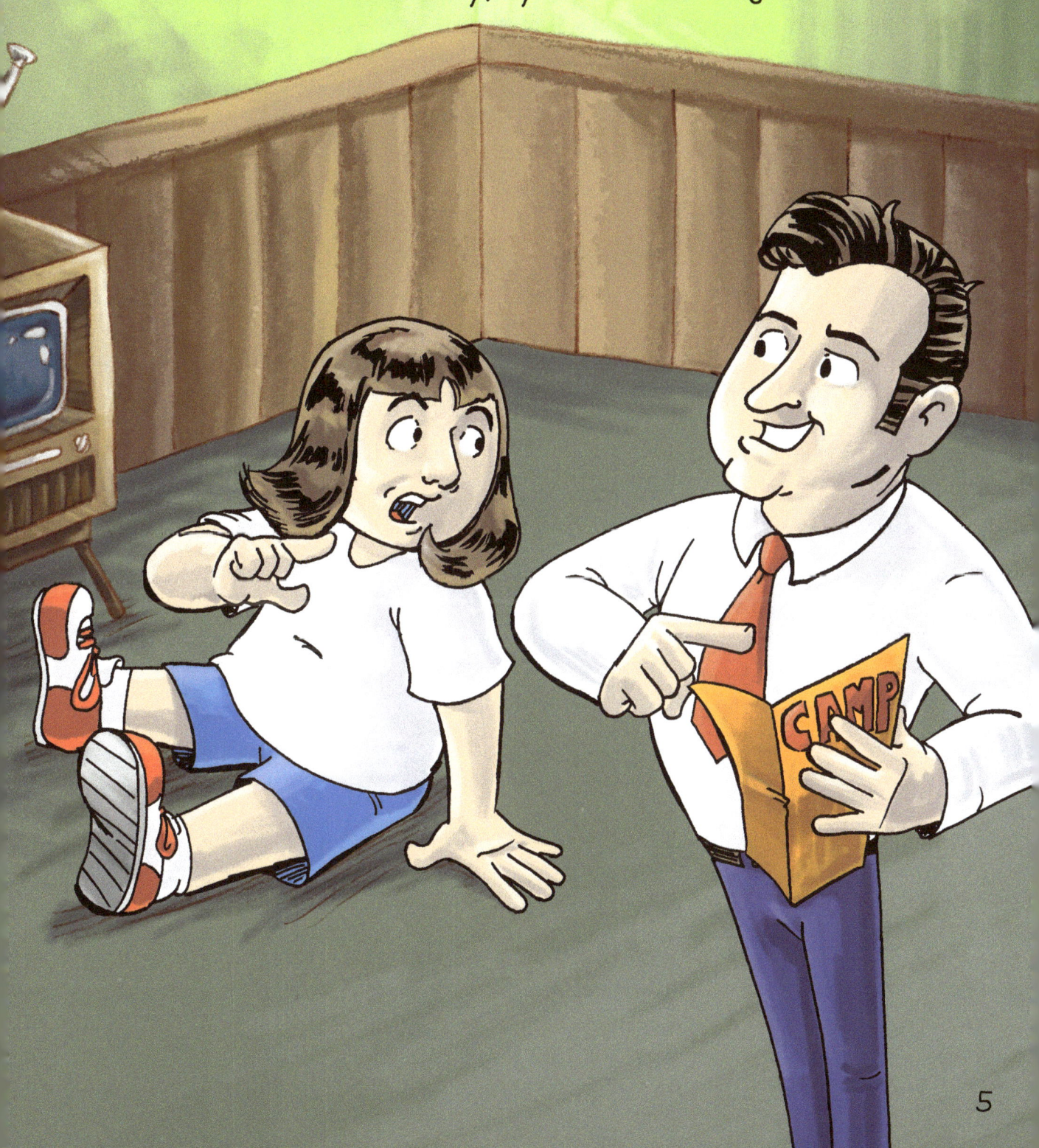

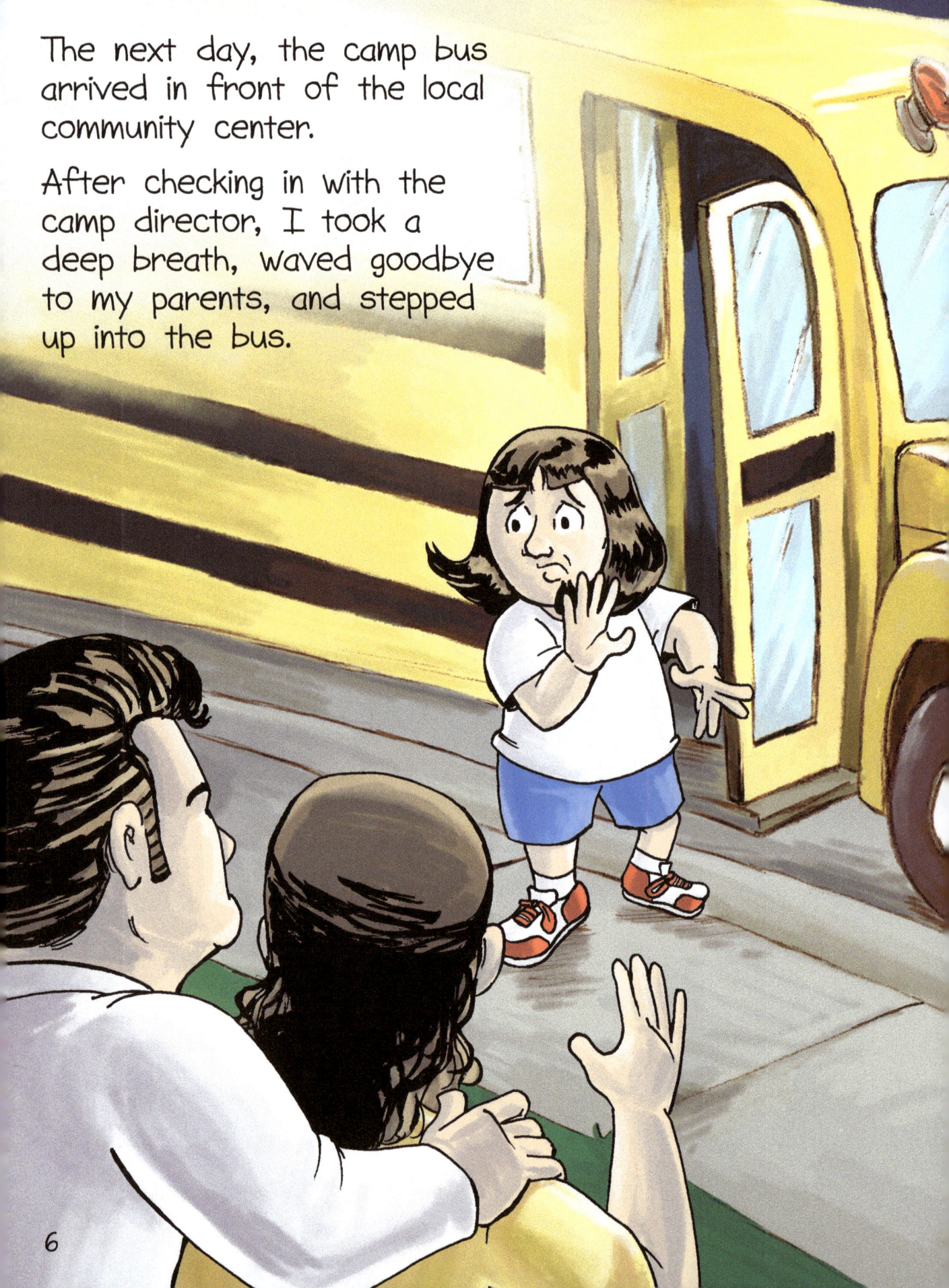

The next day, the camp bus arrived in front of the local community center.

After checking in with the camp director, I took a deep breath, waved goodbye to my parents, and stepped up into the bus.

I sat next to a girl sitting alone.

"I'm Bonnie. What's your name?"

"I'm Roni." We both smiled at the rhyme.

Bonnie said, "This is my first time going to sleep-away camp. I am looking forward to swimming in the lake."

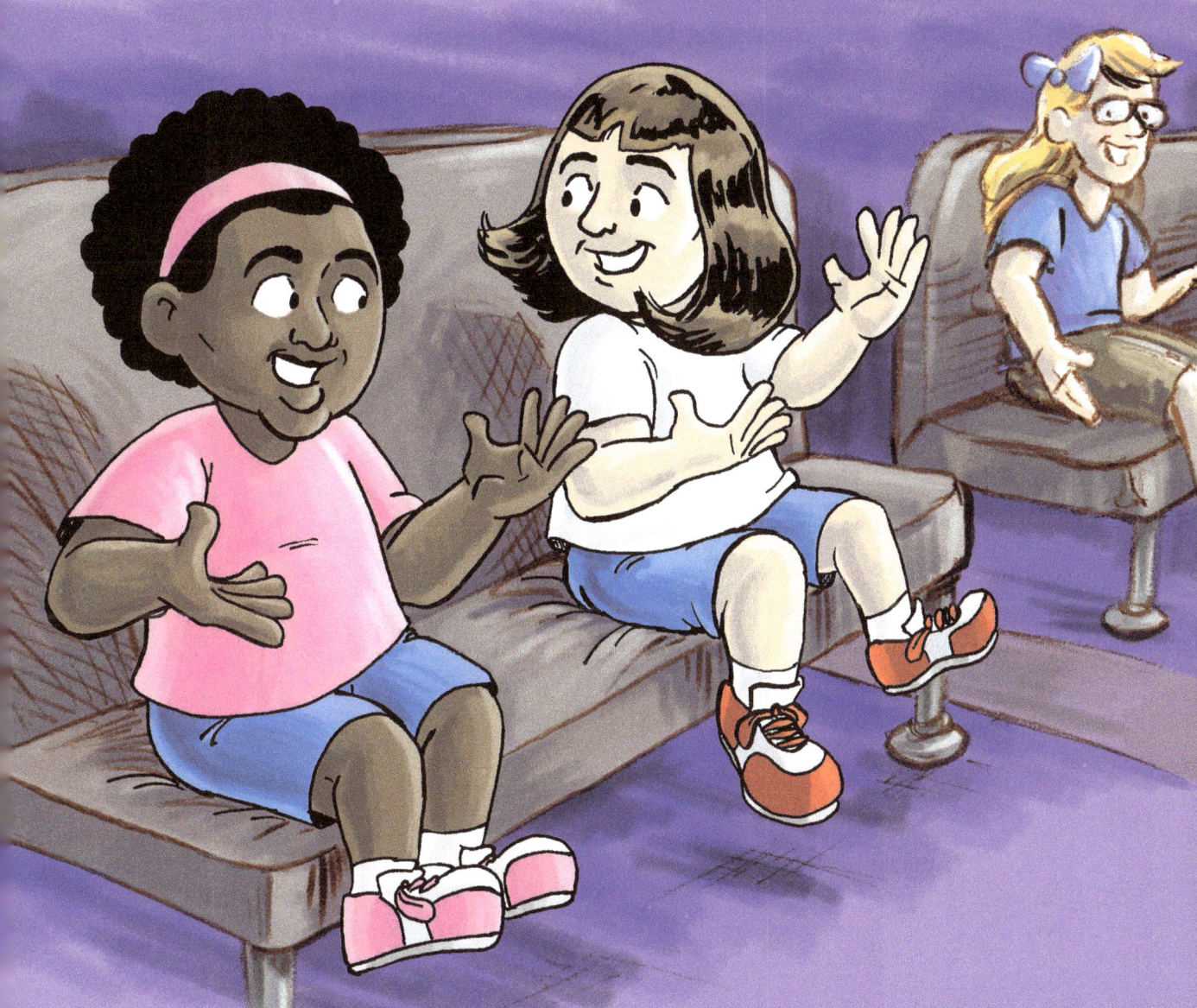

"You're not afraid of being seen in a bathing suit?" I asked.

"No." Bonnie shook her head. "I love to swim."

After a three-hour bus ride, we arrived at camp.

We heard singing:

"Welcome to camp. We're so glad you're here. Have no fear; we're going to have a fun time here. So let's have a big cheer...."

Bonnie and I joined in, "YEAH!!!!"

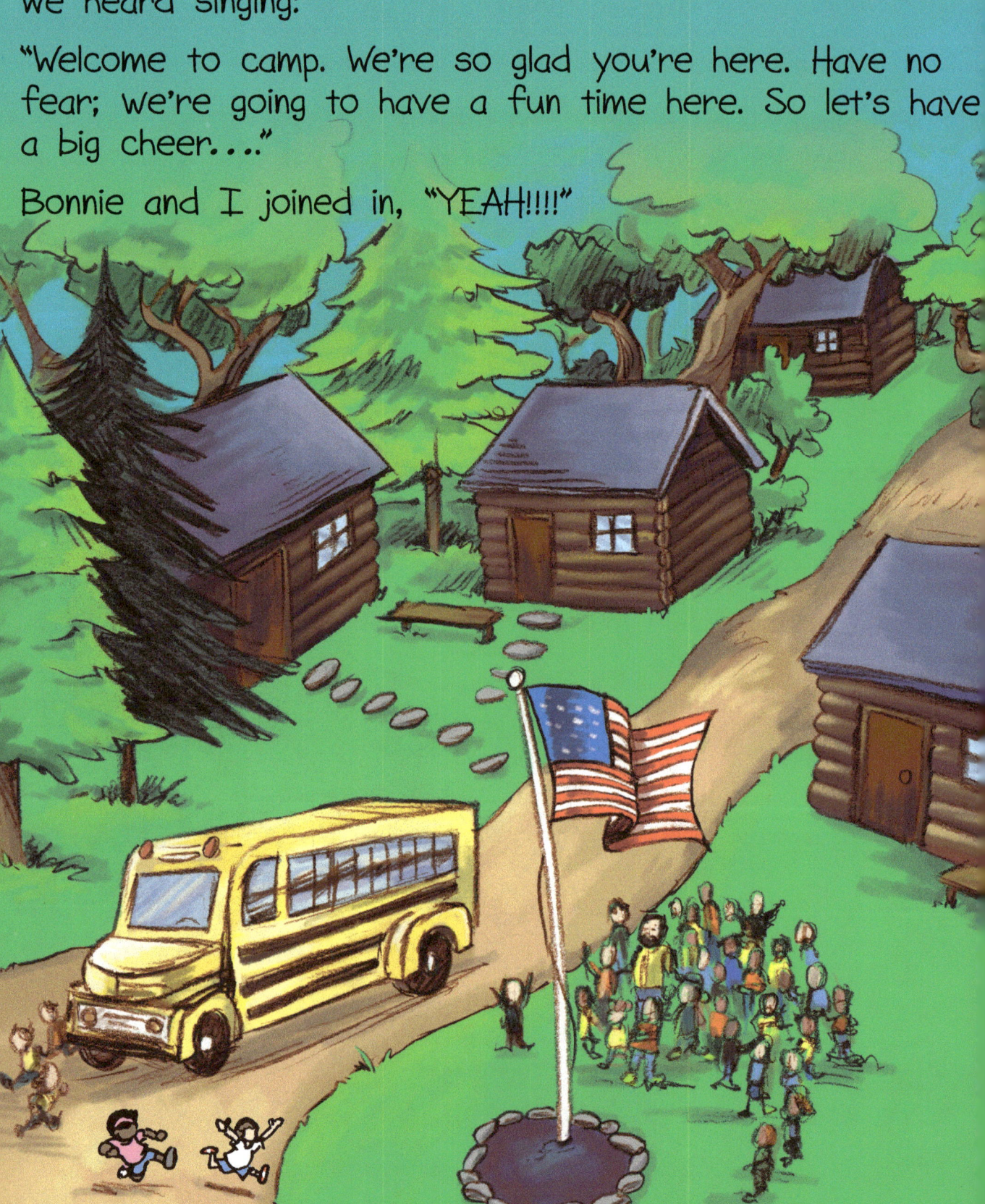

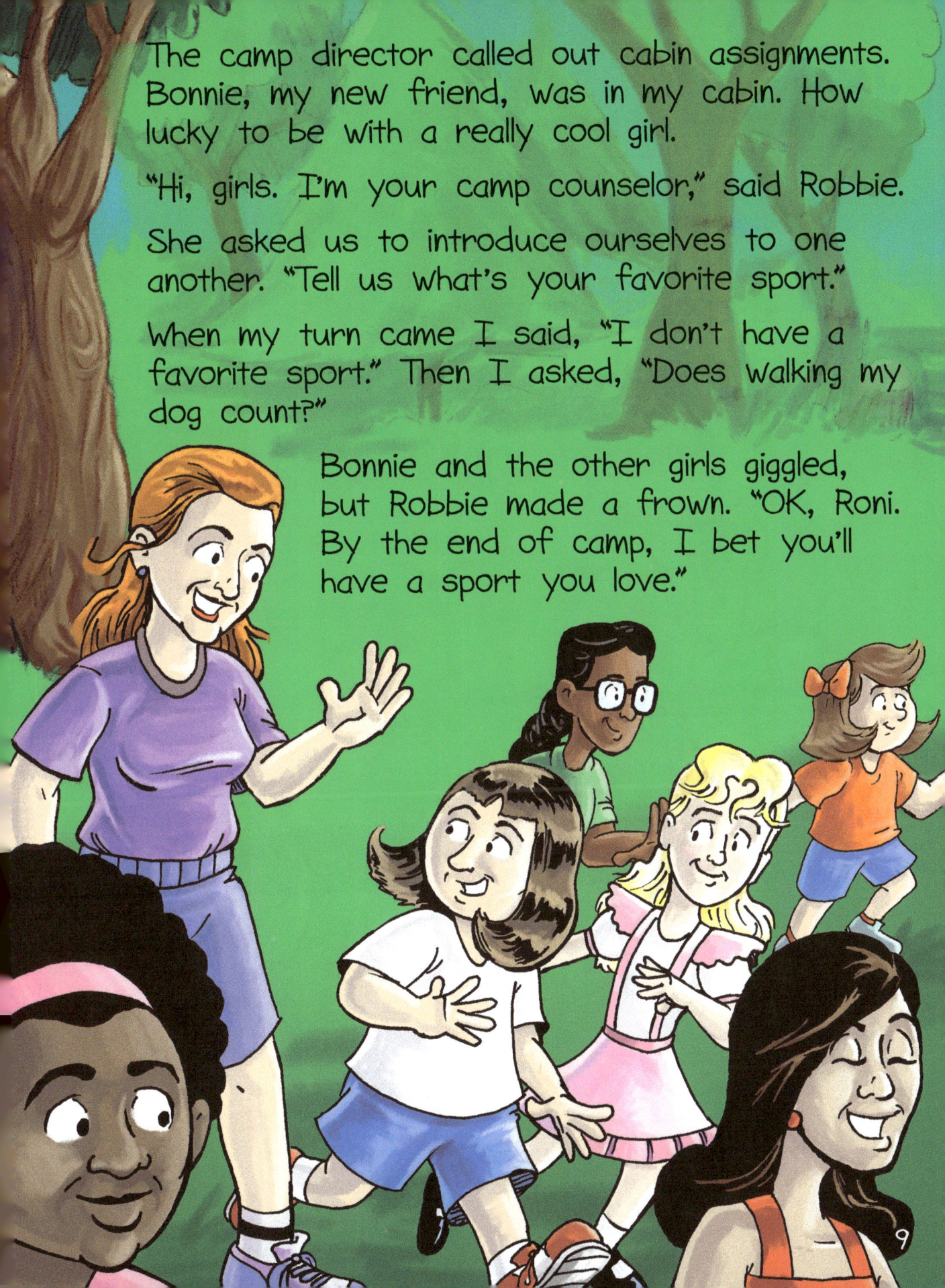

The camp director called out cabin assignments. Bonnie, my new friend, was in my cabin. How lucky to be with a really cool girl.

"Hi, girls. I'm your camp counselor," said Robbie.

She asked us to introduce ourselves to one another. "Tell us what's your favorite sport."

When my turn came I said, "I don't have a favorite sport." Then I asked, "Does walking my dog count?"

Bonnie and the other girls giggled, but Robbie made a frown. "OK, Roni. By the end of camp, I bet you'll have a sport you love."

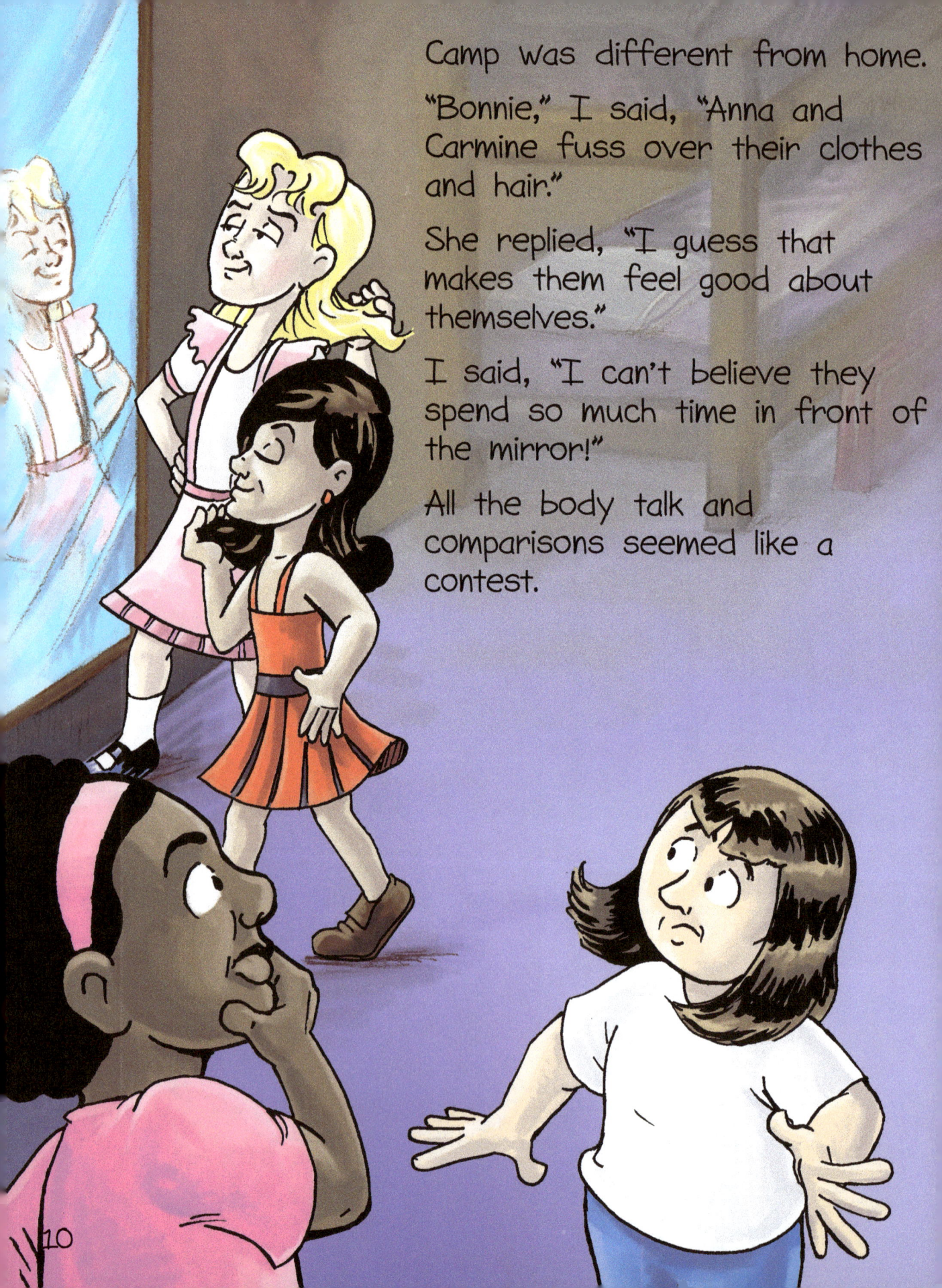

Camp was different from home.

"Bonnie," I said, "Anna and Carmine fuss over their clothes and hair."

She replied, "I guess that makes them feel good about themselves."

I said, "I can't believe they spend so much time in front of the mirror!"

All the body talk and comparisons seemed like a contest.

Sonja, a quiet girl in my cabin, made the most beautiful beaded bracelets during arts and crafts time. One bracelet she made had an unusual pattern.

I told Sonja, "I love this bracelet."

Sonja picked up the bracelet and said, "Roni, I want you to have this as a friendship bracelet."

"Thanks, Sonja!" I said.

From that day on, Sonja and I were best buddies.

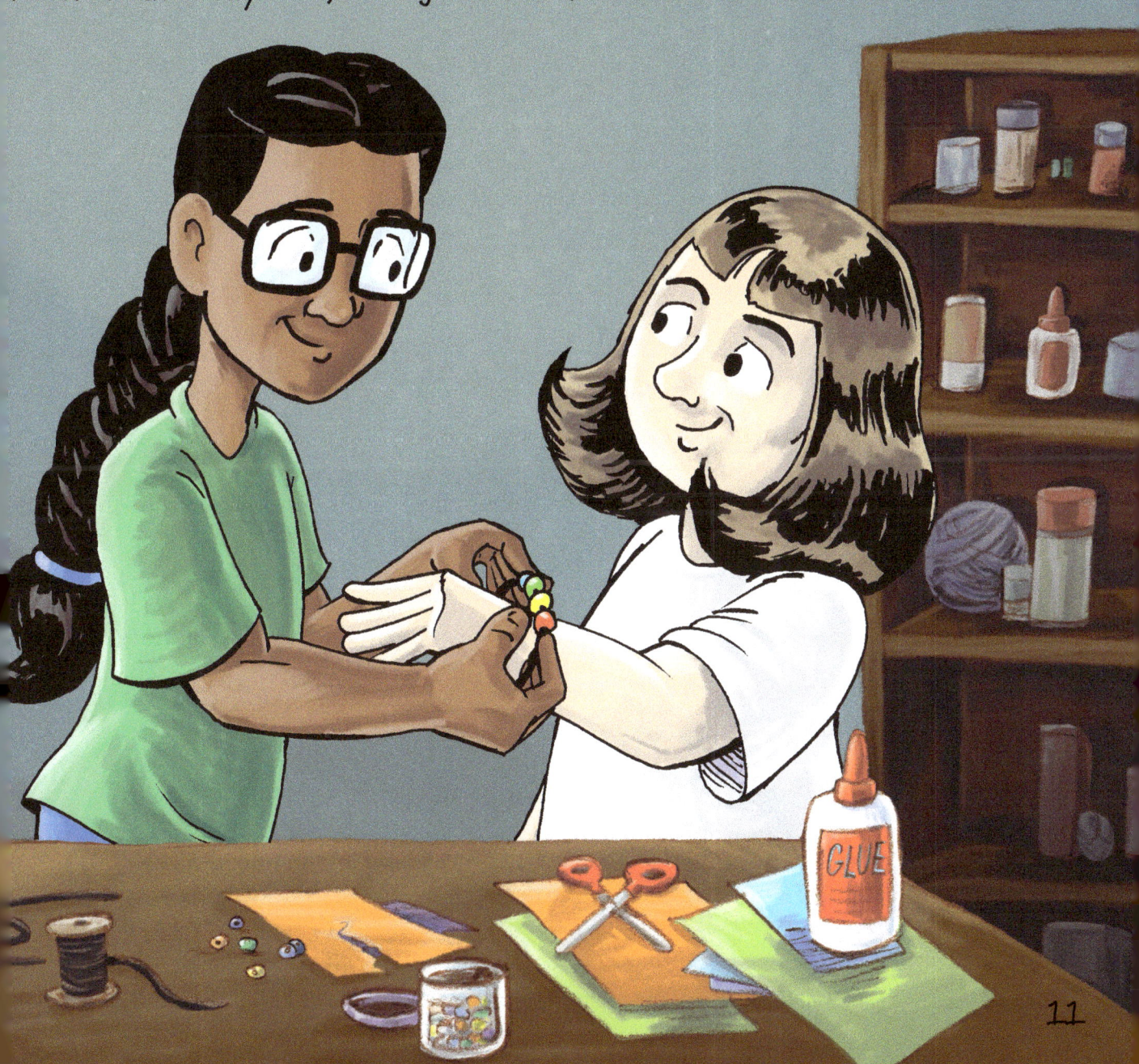

The mess hall, where we ate our meals, was another new experience for me. Each cabin sat together at long tables.

Food in the mess hall was served family style. That means large plates and bowls of food were brought to the table for everyone to share.

We even drank something called "bug juice." It was very sweet. I thought by the way it tasted, bug juice must be loaded with lots of sugar.

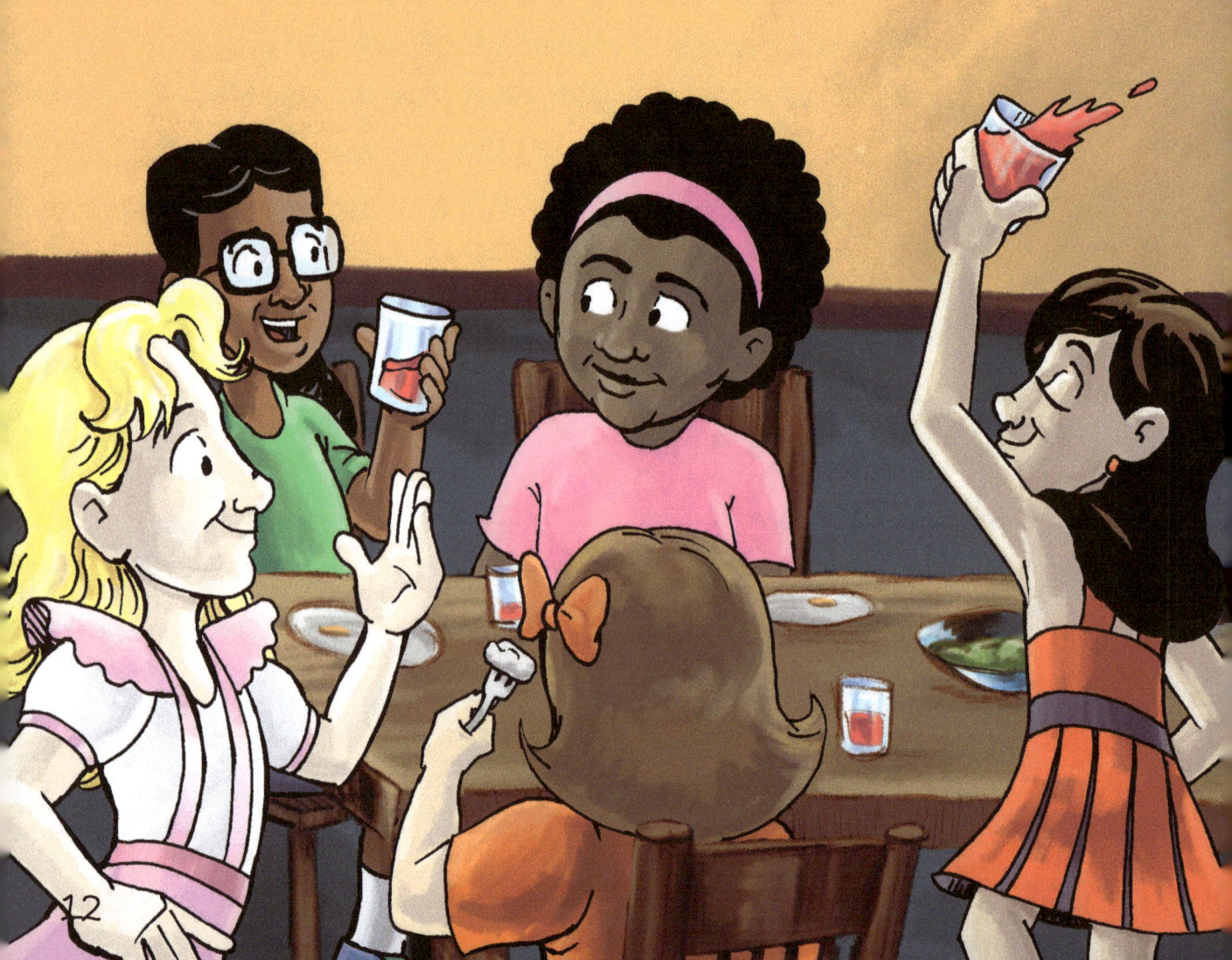

At mealtime, Robbie watched over me like a mother hen. I felt so uncomfortable.

One time at dinner, Robbie looked at me sternly. "Roni, you need to put that spoonful of mashed potatoes back in the bowl. You've had enough!"

I slid down in my chair, wishing I could disappear.

Robbie monitored not only what I ate but also how much I ate. I didn't like it!

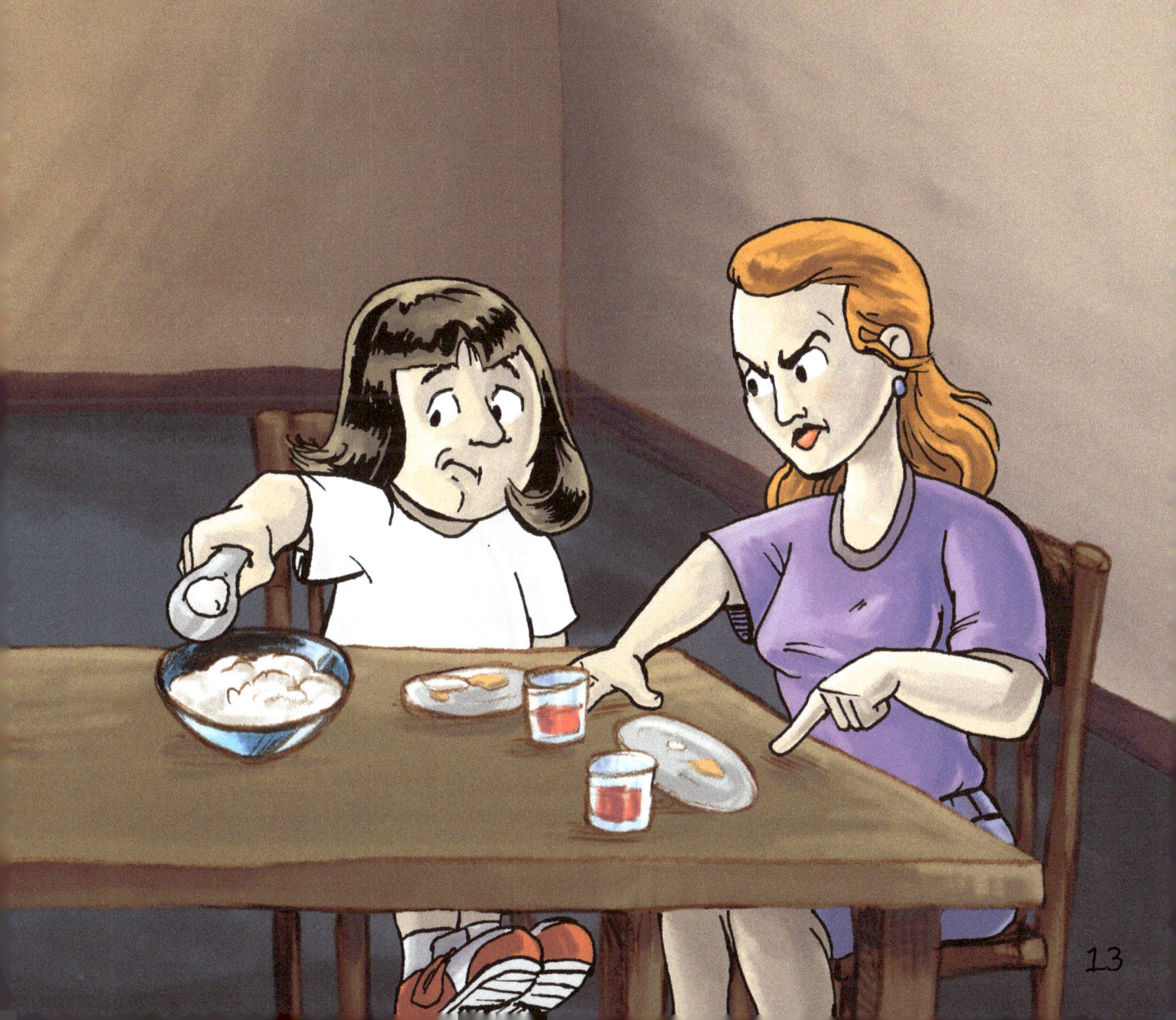

Sports were a big part of camp life.

To my surprise, swimming was the sport I liked best.

The swimming instructor helped me learn to swim. He lifted me up in the water with one hand under my belly and said, "Kick, Roni, kick." Then he said, "Now, use your arms, Roni, and make overhead strokes, like you're paddling the water."

I tried and tried again. The more I did it, the better I got.

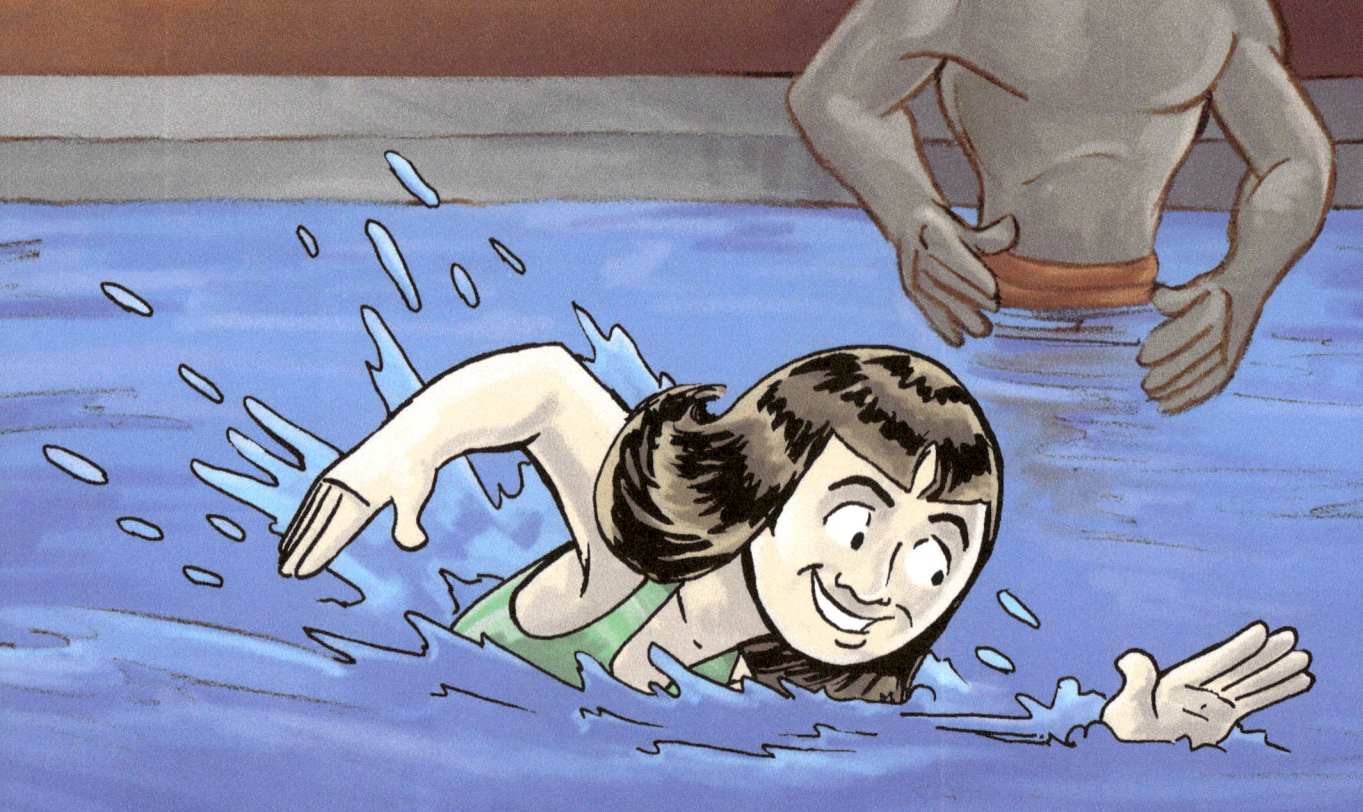

Despite my efforts, Robbie made my life miserable at camp.

On the softball field, she told me, "Roni, you need to run faster."

Even when we walked from one activity to another, Robbie held my hand so I wouldn't lag behind the group.

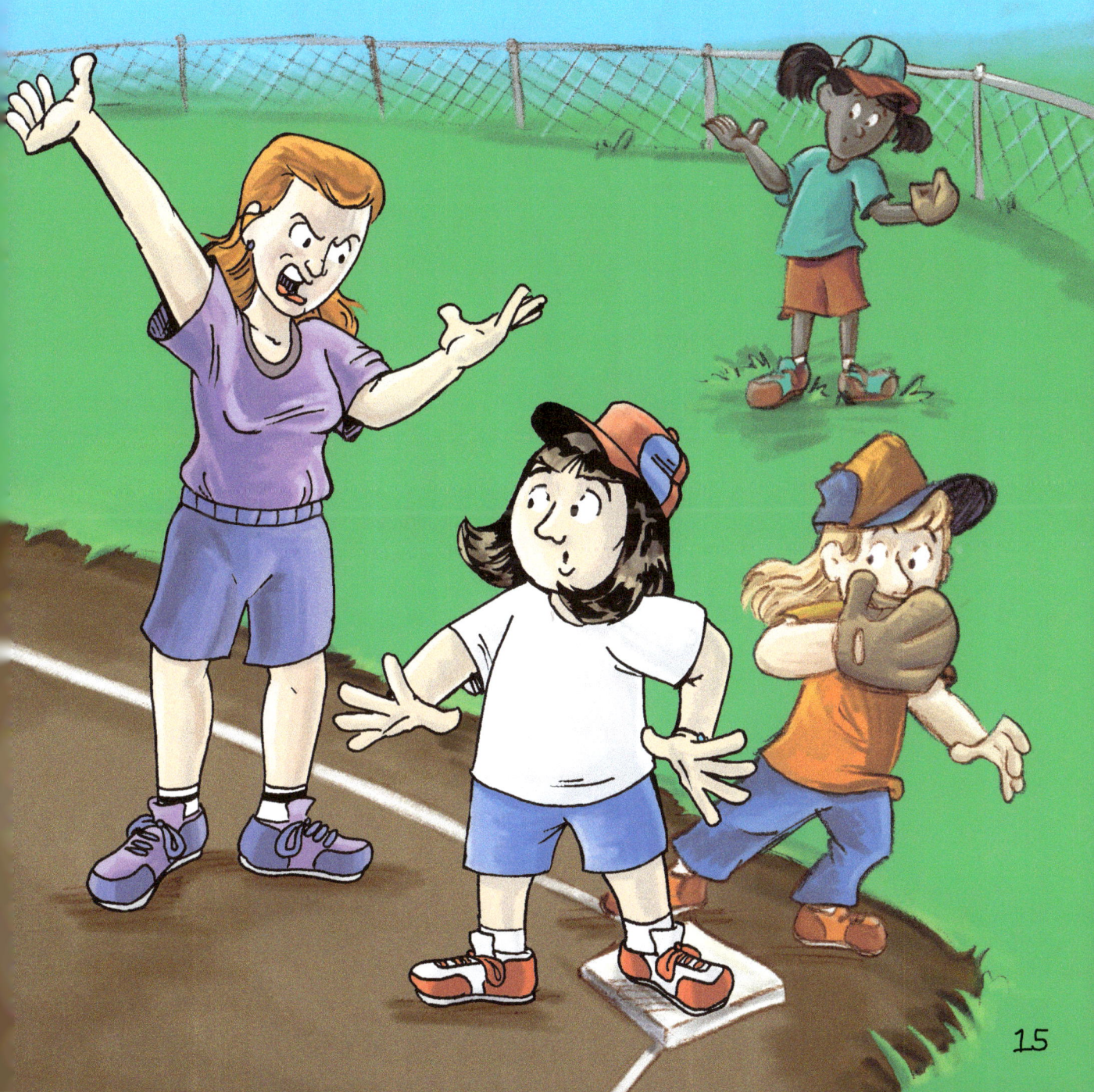

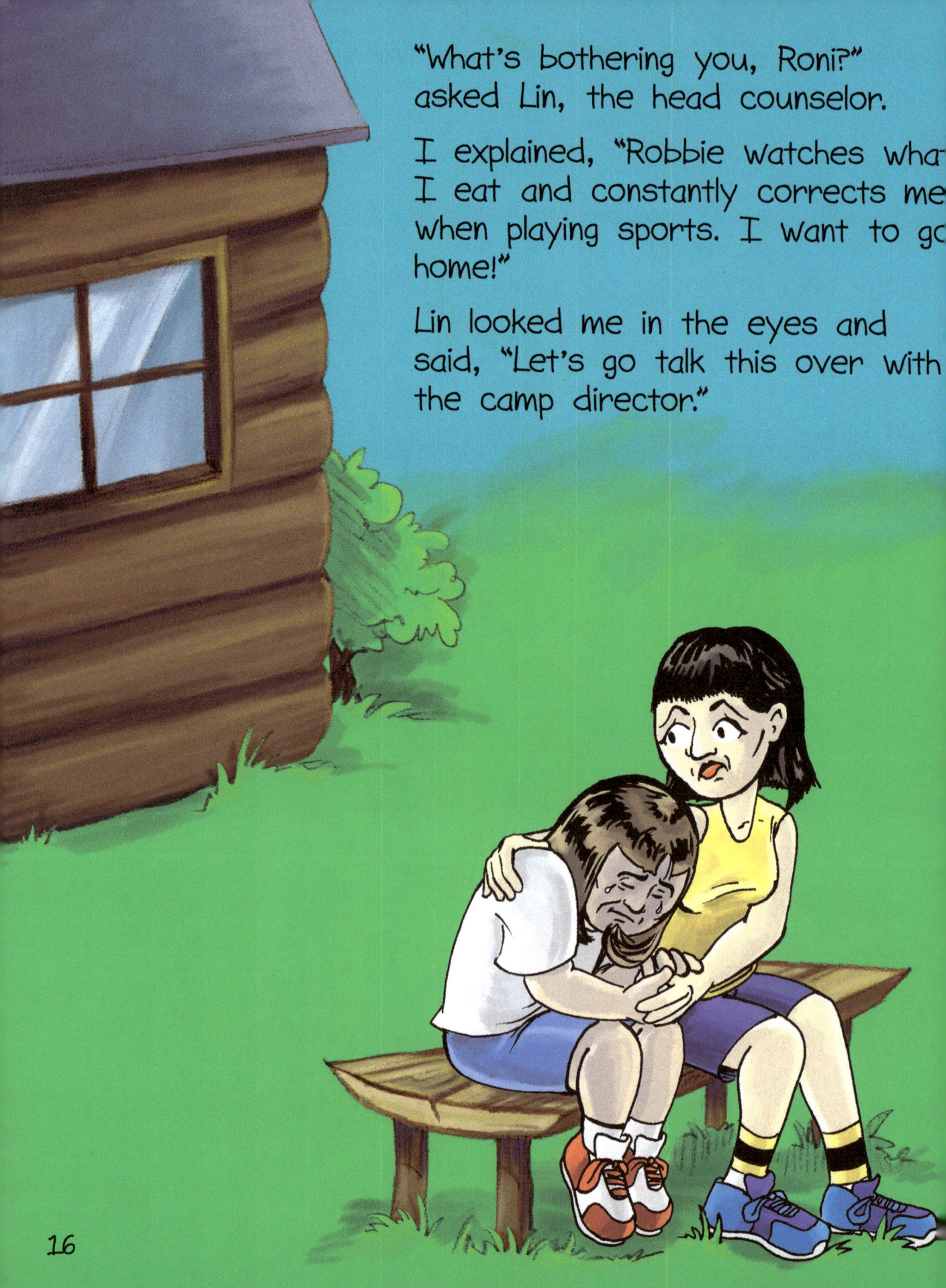

"What's bothering you, Roni?" asked Lin, the head counselor.

I explained, "Robbie watches what I eat and constantly corrects me when playing sports. I want to go home!"

Lin looked me in the eyes and said, "Let's go talk this over with the camp director."

The camp director said, "Roni, we want you to have a positive camp experience. Let me see what we can do."

I asked, "Can I call home?"

On the telephone, I told my mom what was going on.

Mom said, "Roni, I understand you're having a difficult time. The camp director will handle it."

"Don't give up," Mom insisted.

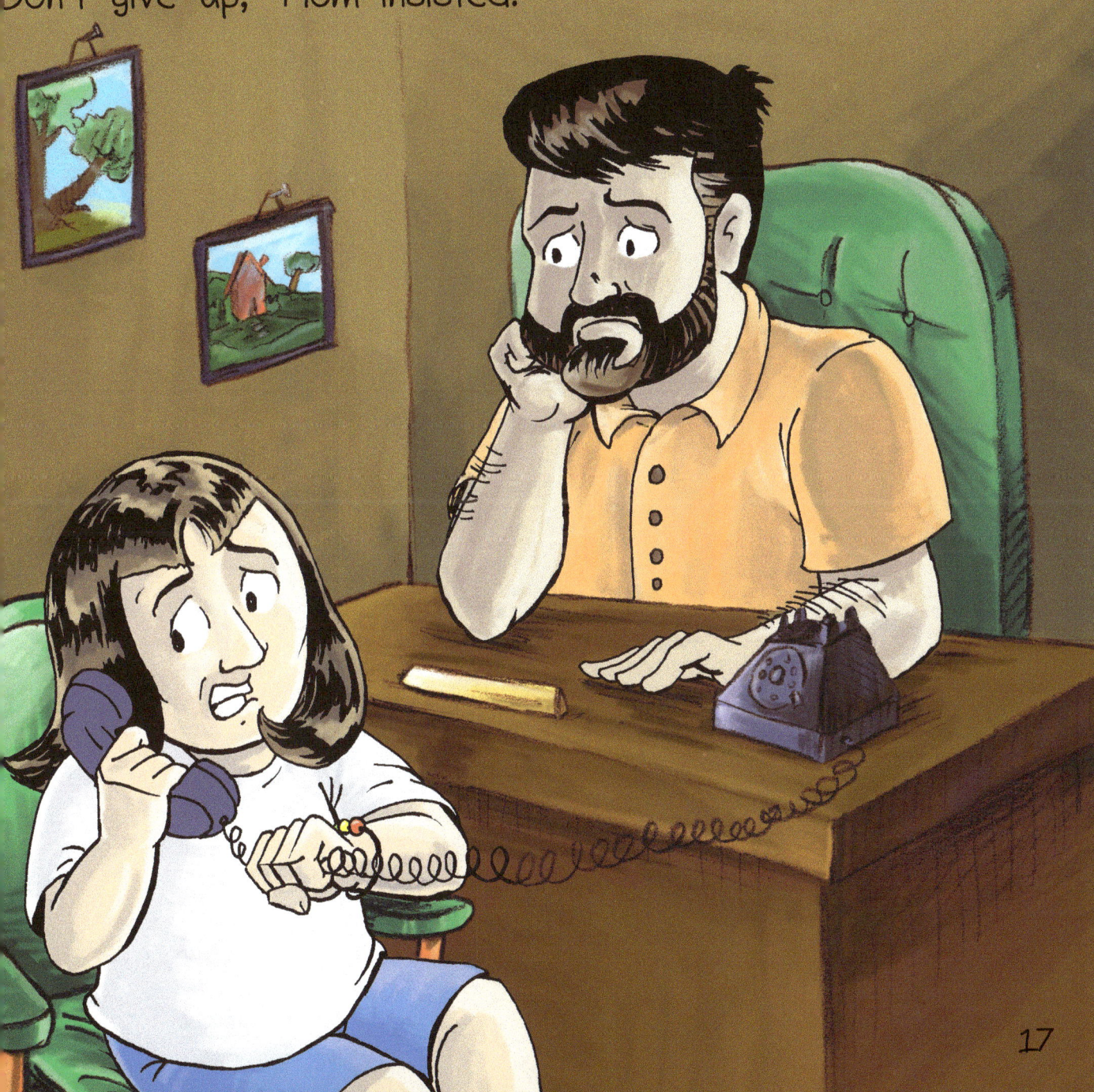

Lin and I walked back to the cabin together. The girls from the cabin gathered around me.

Bonnie said, "I'm sorry you feel so bad, Roni. I would miss you if you went home before camp was over. You are my best friend at camp."

Sonja chimed in, "Roni, who would I talk to during arts and crafts? Who would make me laugh?"

Anna and Carmine whispered to me, "We'll stop telling you what to wear and how to dress. Just stay. Please...."

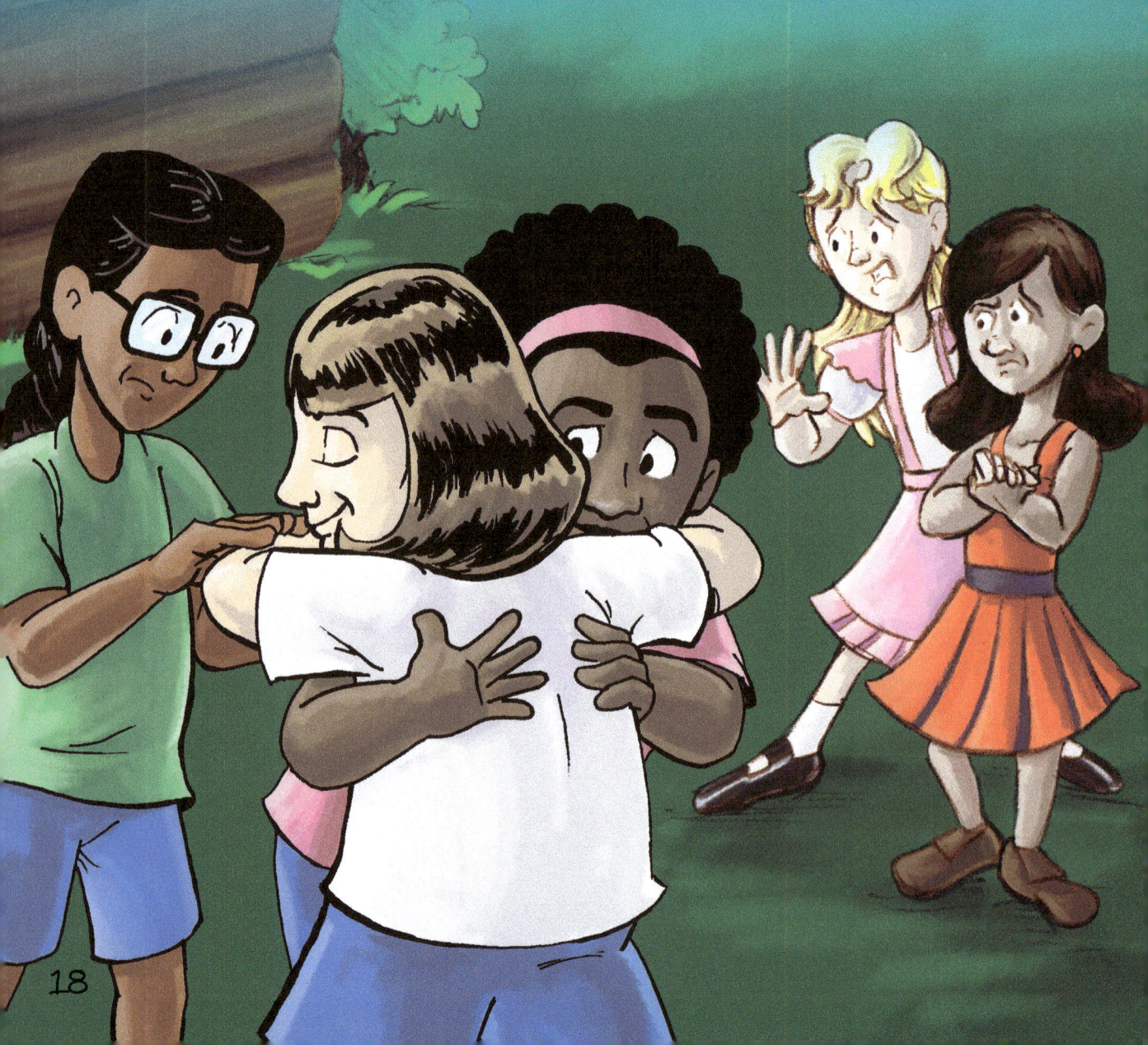

Later Robbie came back to the cabin. "Roni, I'm sorry I picked on you. I was not considerate of your feelings."

I just stared at her.

"Roni, I was like you as a young girl. I learned from the camp director it is best for me to be a good role model for you and the other girls."

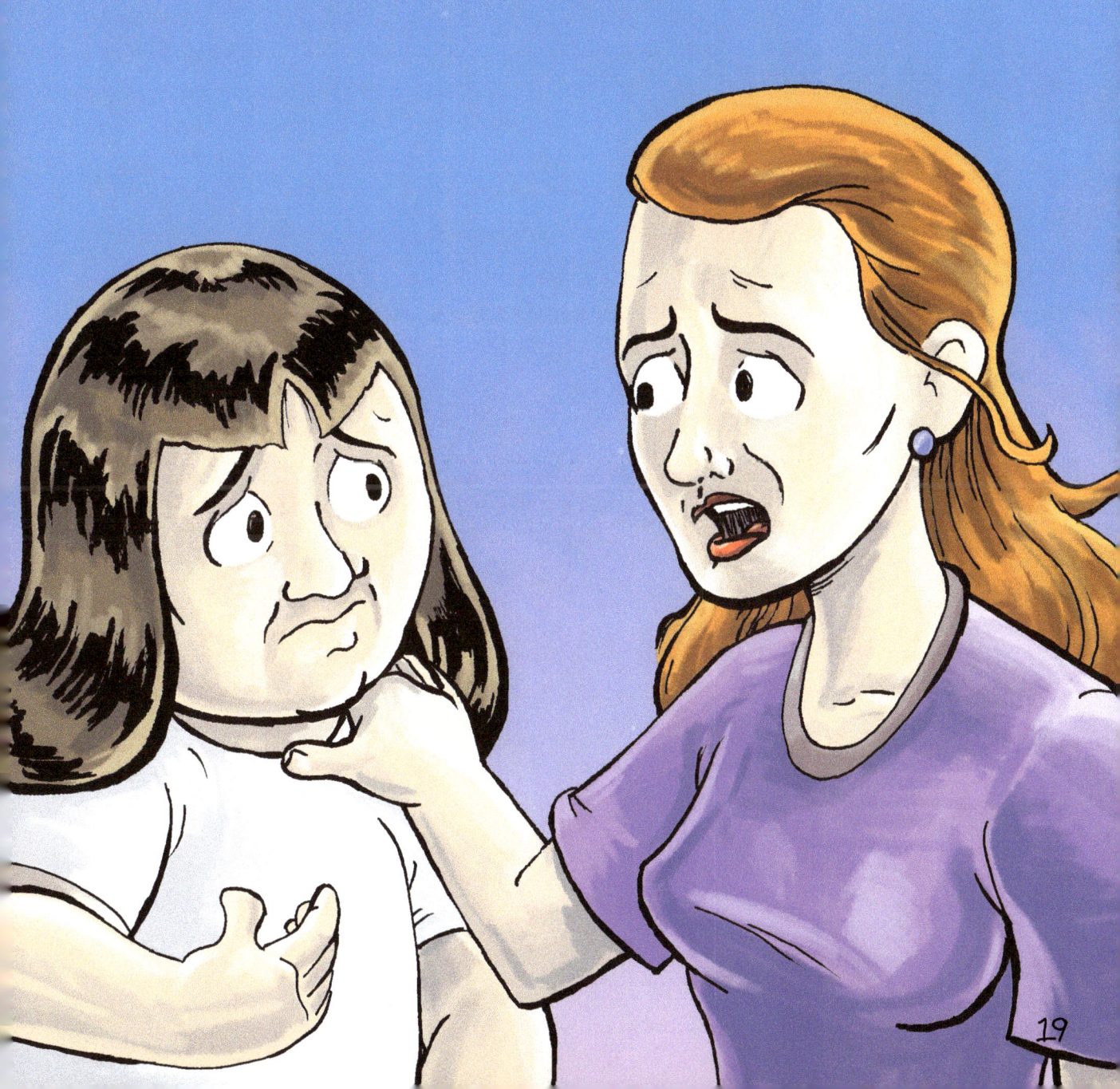

A few days later the camp director told everyone, "I am pleased to announce the formation of the first Camp Wellness Council."

He said, "Camp is a place to promote health and learn positive life skills. Each camper possesses special strengths and unique qualities."

I was surprised--Robbie and I were asked to participate on the Council.

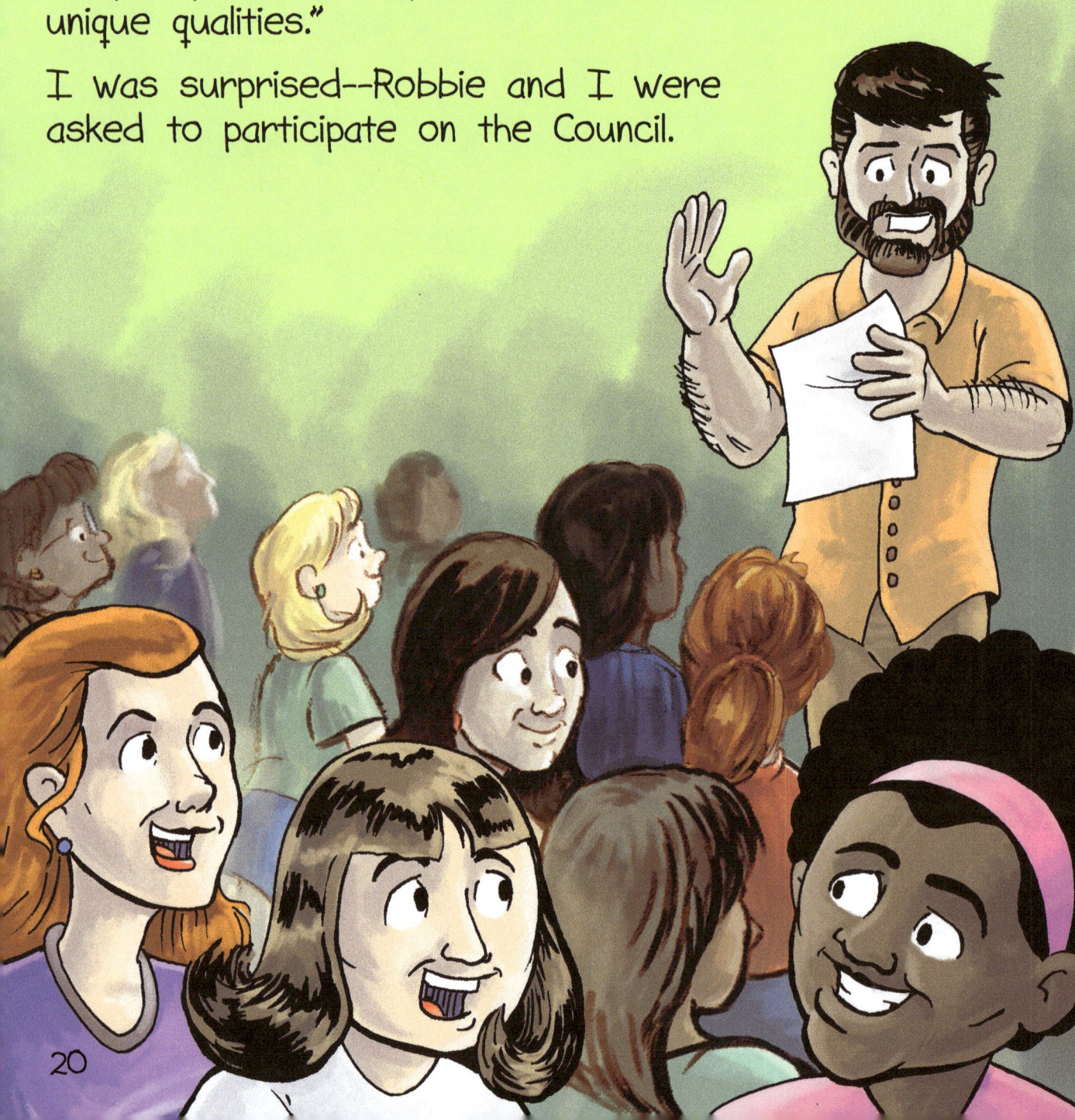

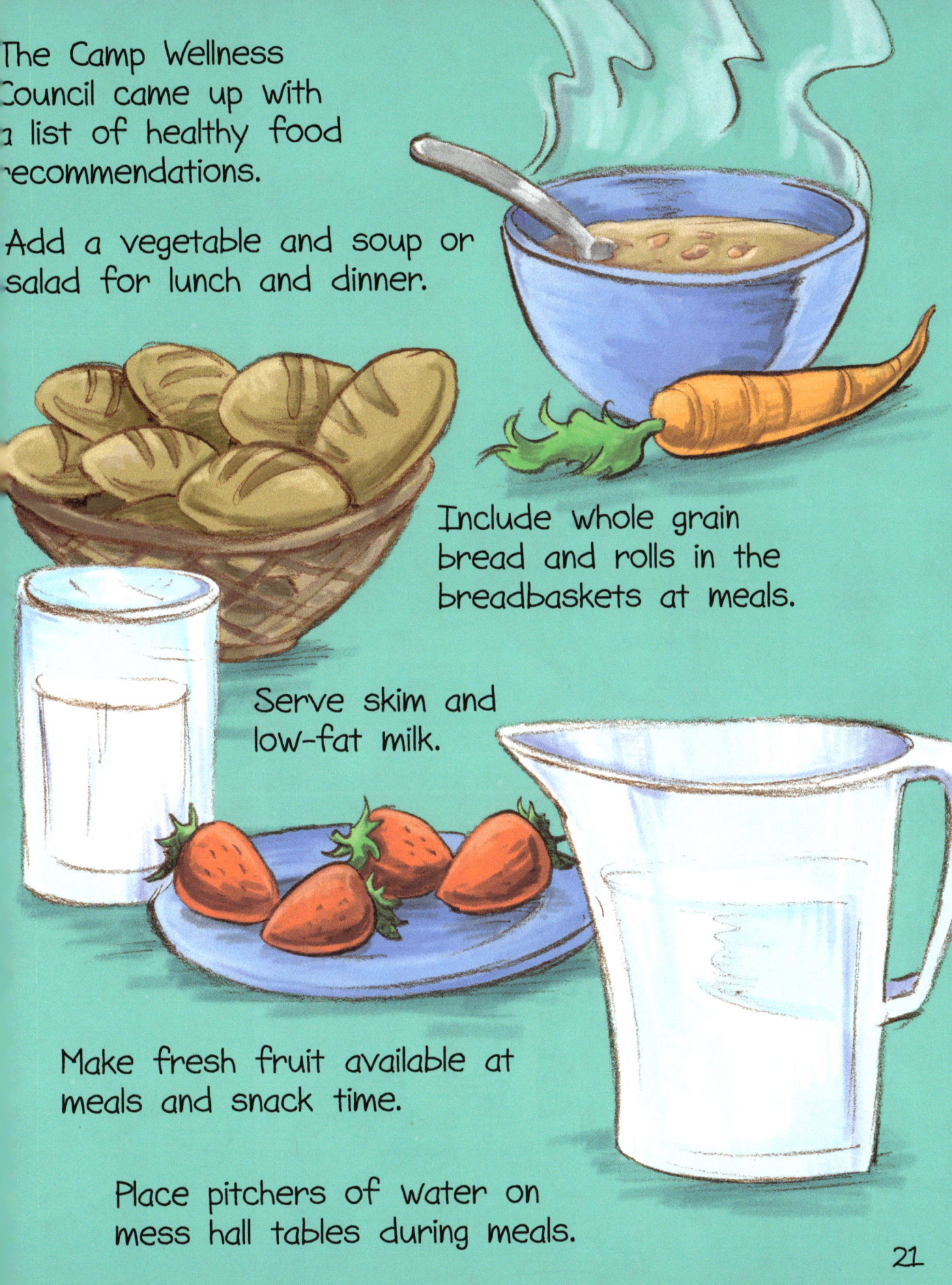

The Camp Wellness Council came up with a list of healthy food recommendations.

Add a vegetable and soup or salad for lunch and dinner.

Include whole grain bread and rolls in the breadbaskets at meals.

Serve skim and low-fat milk.

Make fresh fruit available at meals and snack time.

Place pitchers of water on mess hall tables during meals.

Members of the Camp Wellness Council began introducing food and nutrition tips for campers.

Tip #1: Brighten your plate with colorful fruits and vegetables; they provide important vitamins and minerals and are low in calories.

Tip #2: Try to drink water when thirsty instead of sugary bug juice.

Tip #3: Tonight is movie night. Plain popcorn is a healthy whole grain snack choice.

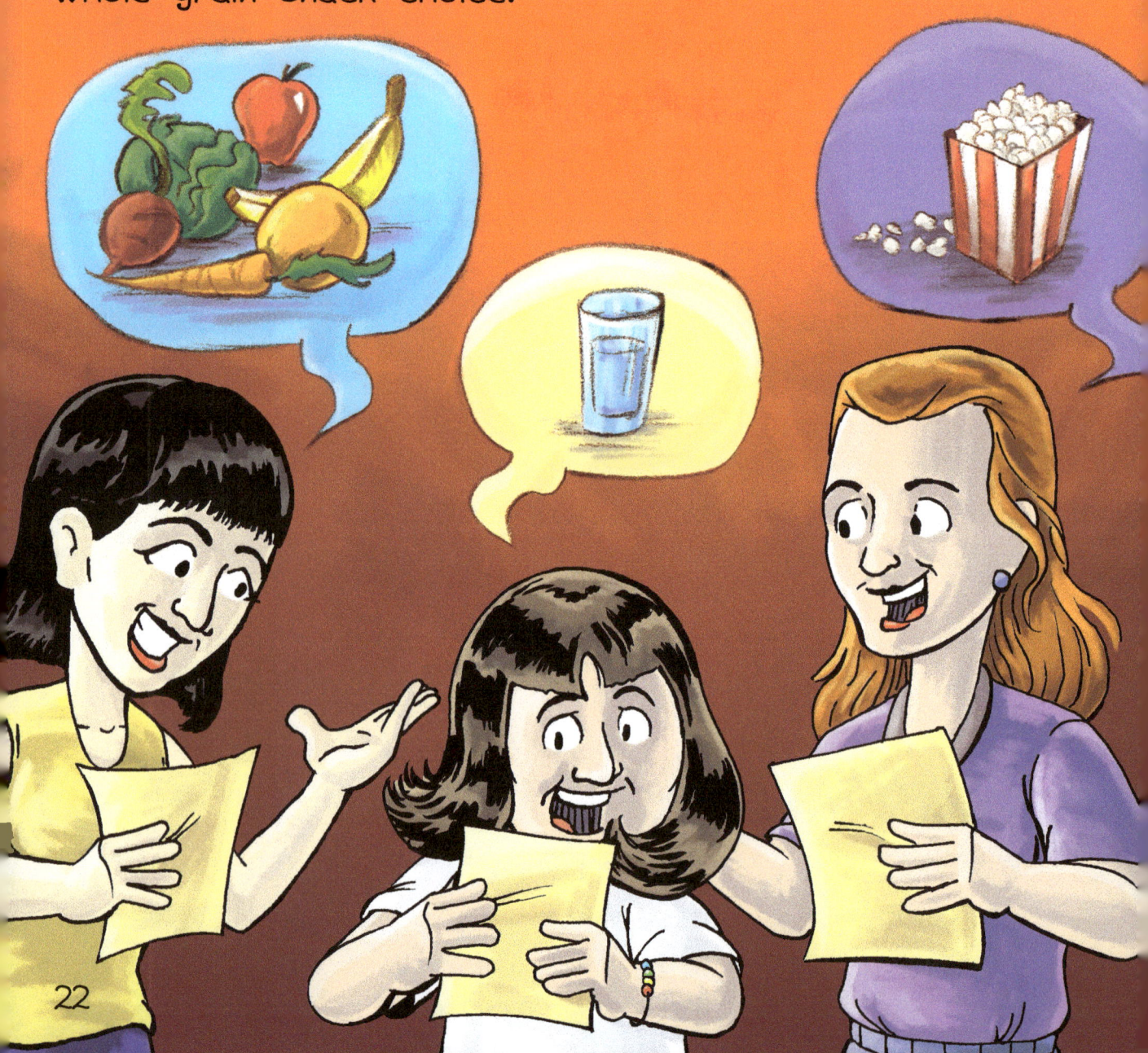

The Camp Wellness Council came up with another great idea--starting a vegetable and herb garden.

Jin announced, "We are looking for campers to set up the first camp garden. You need to be willing to get your hands and clothes dirty as we clear the field."

She explained, "It's too late this summer to plant vegetables, but next year staff members will get the garden going early in the season."

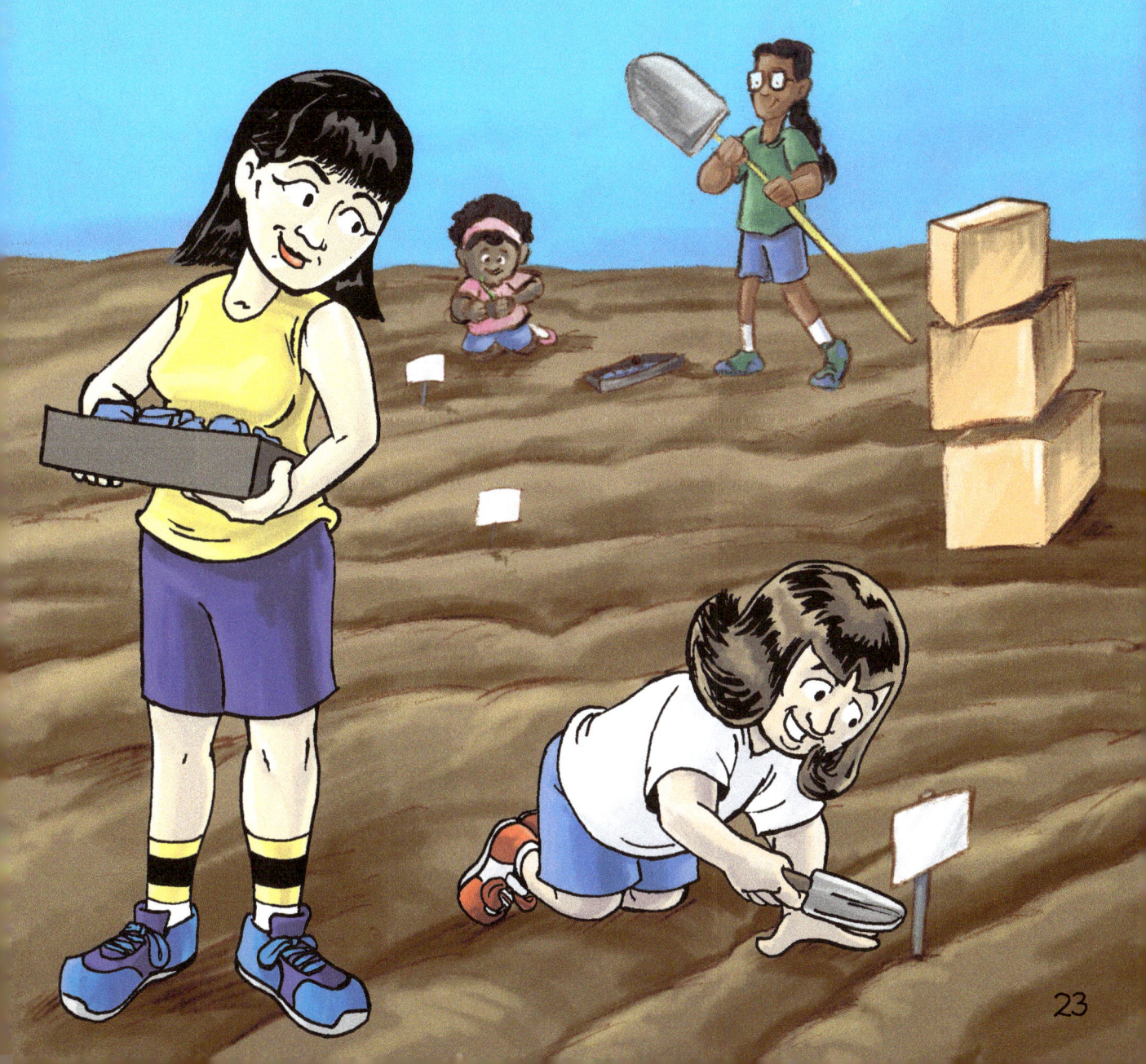

A camp snack station was set up outside the mess hall. The camp cook gave us fun and simple foods to prepare during the afternoon rest period.

One recipe was hummus with fresh cut-up vegetables and whole grain crackers. Delicious!

For campfires, we roasted marshmallows with pieces of fresh fruit on a long stick. I enjoyed making the treats and eating them!

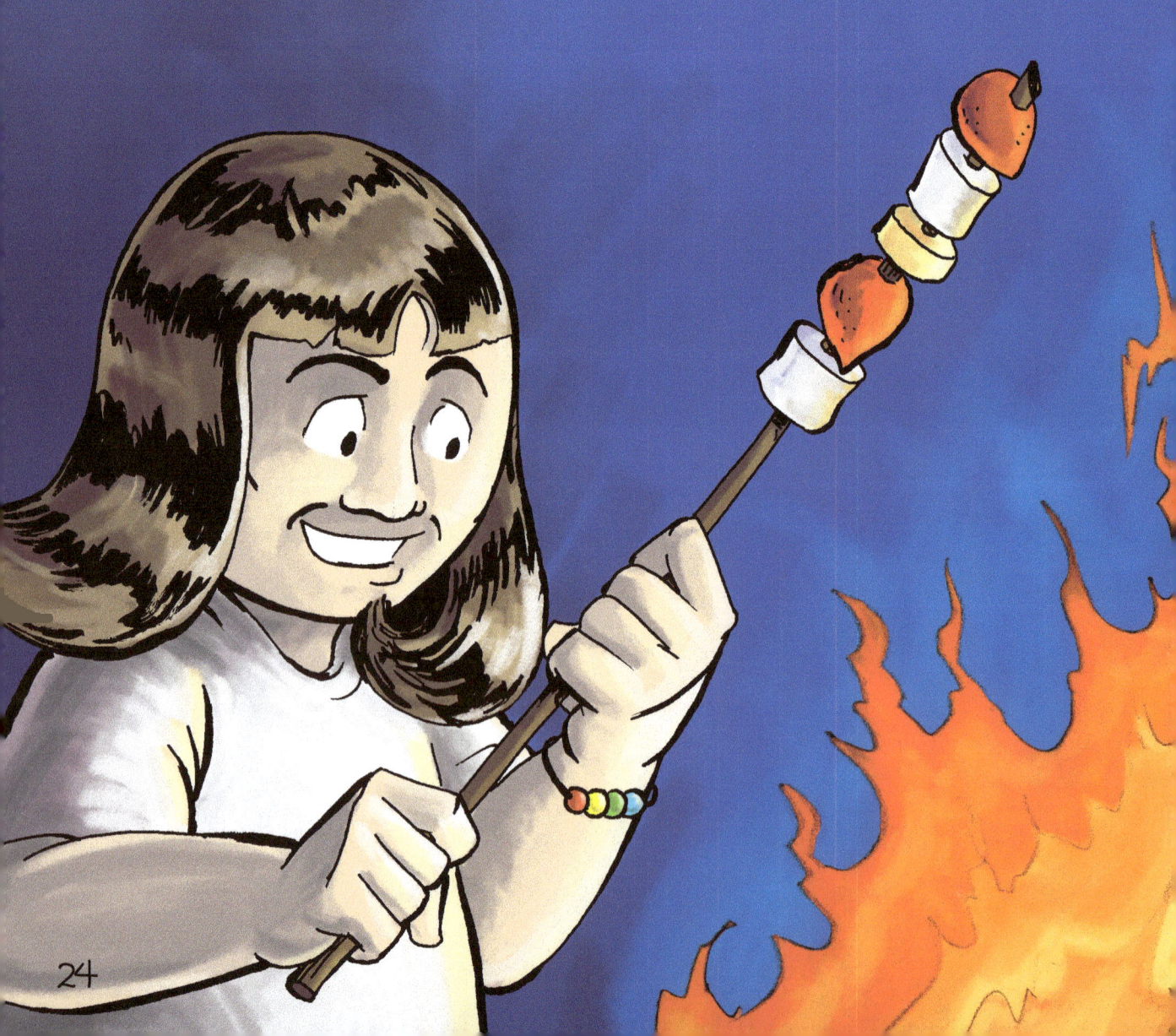

The end of camp was near. It was time for the final sports competition.

Half the camp was on the red team; the other half was on the blue team.

I woke up one morning to find a blue string attached to my bed.

Robbie said, "Roni, you are on the blue team along with Bonnie and Sonja. The other girls in the cabin have been assigned to the red team."

I chose swimming, softball, and volleyball as my blue team events.

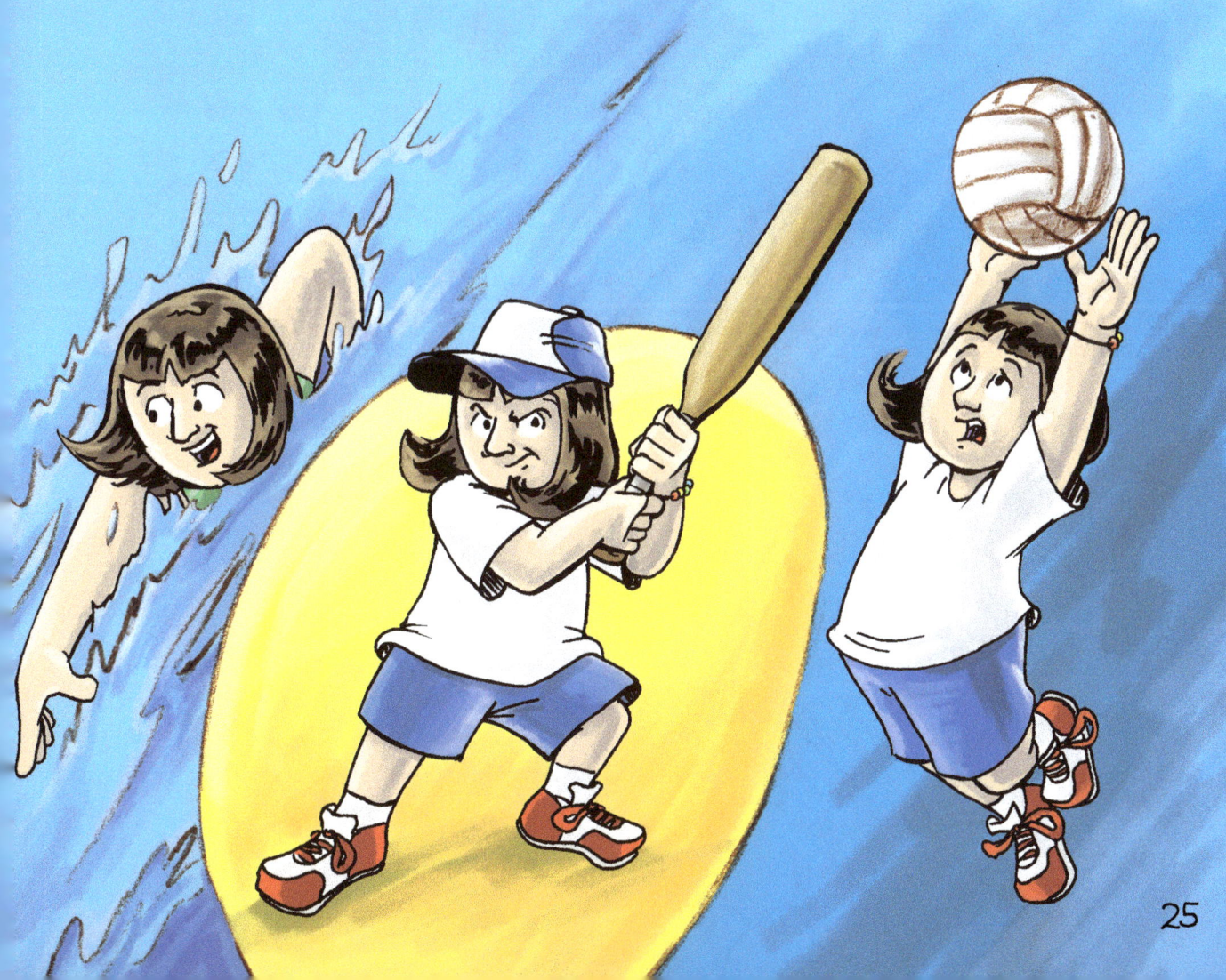

The blue team lost. I was very disappointed, but I still had lots of fun being part of a team.

At the awards ceremony, the camp director called out, "Roni, I am pleased to name you the most improved swimmer for your age group." He shook my hand and pinned a beautiful ribbon to my camp shirt.

Next, Lin got up to speak. "I want to thank the Camp Wellness Council. Great strides were made this summer to create a healthy camp environment for now and for future summer sessions."

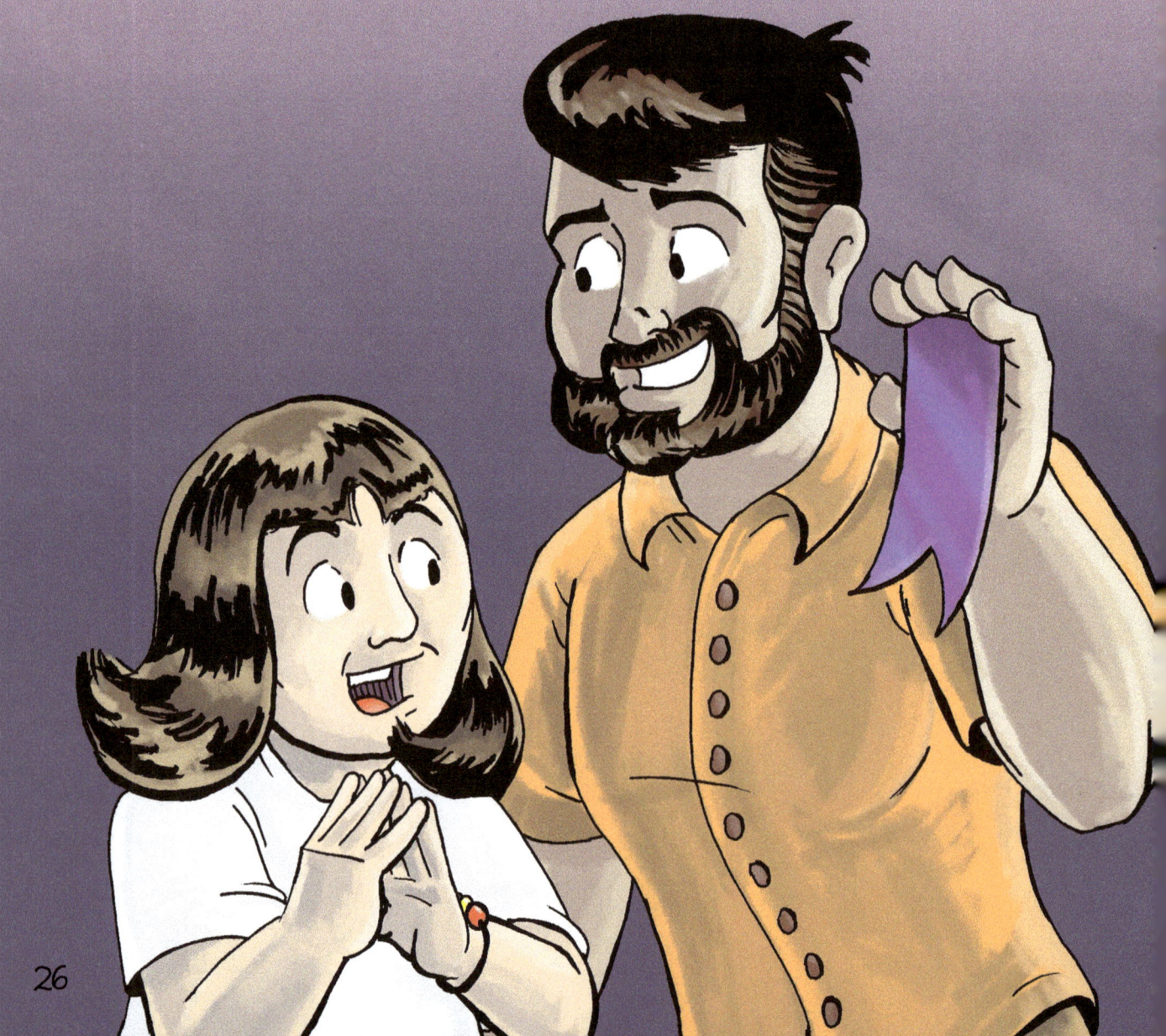

Before leaving camp for home, Robbie took me aside.

She said, "No matter how much I may think I know, there is always more to learn. One size doesn't fit all. I will never forget this summer and being your camp counselor."

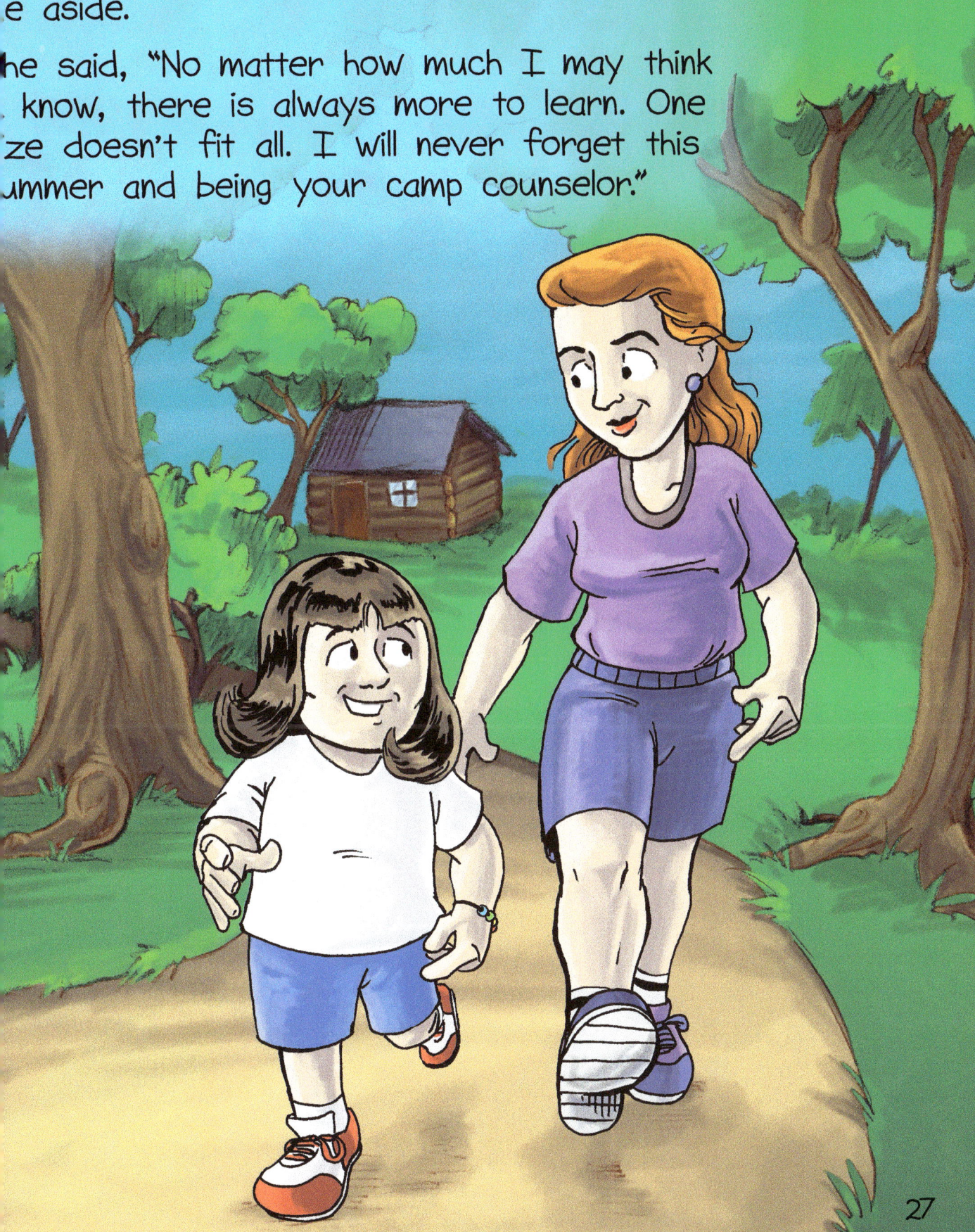

Dad was right. Going to camp was great, although it did take some adjustment!

I love my new friends and feel more confident about myself.

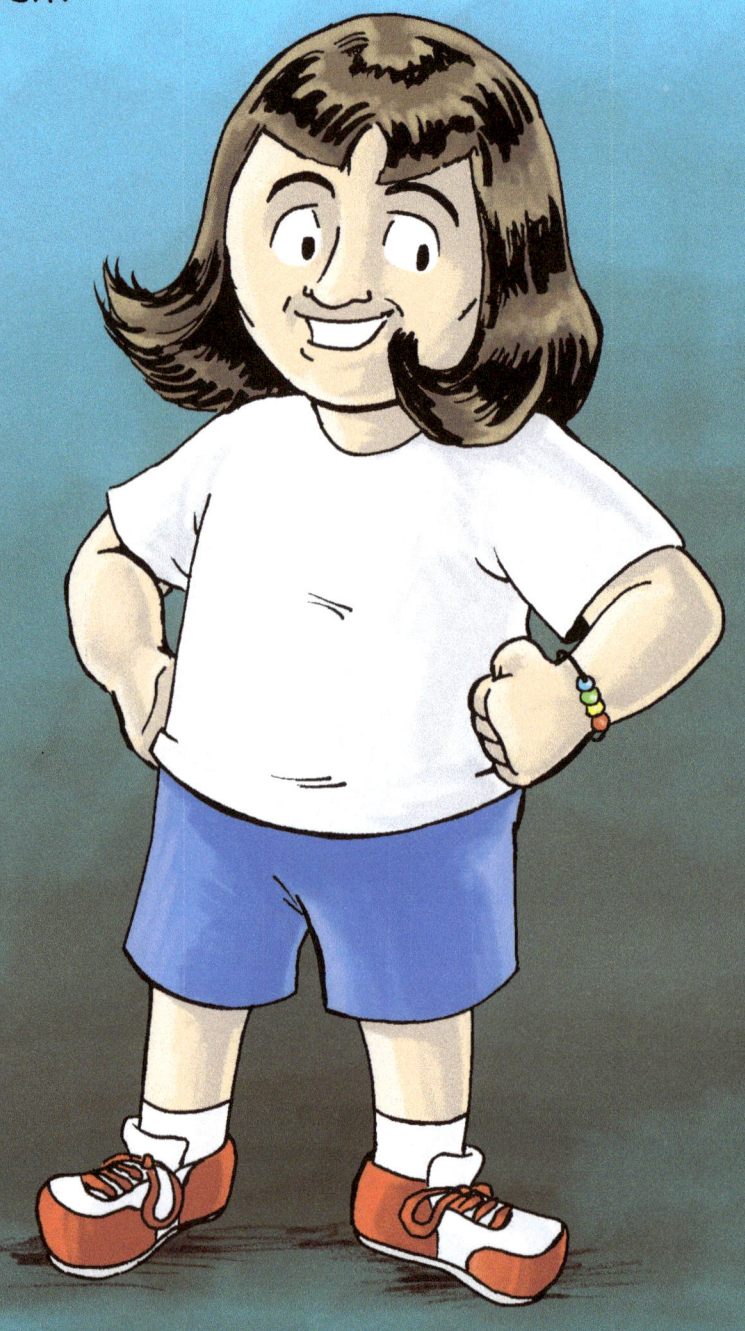

My new motto is, "Doing is freeing. Free to be the best that I can be."

Afterword

Summer camp provides an opportunity for children to learn, grow, and mature while confronting the world, quite possibly for the first time on their own. Its unique experiences and landscapes teach respect for nature; invite growth of knowledge, skill, and spirit; and afford children the chance to acquire valuable lifestyle practices for health and wellness.

Many children today are overweight or obese. Camp can be part of the solution to the childhood obesity challenge. Whether it is day camp or sleep-away camp, one week long or several weeks, summer camp offers children a structured environment with social, physical, and recreational activities when school is not in session. Let's make summer camp, with supportive health promotion policies and personnel, a reality for all children.

Online Helpful Resources

Kids Eat Right

www.eatright.org/kids

Let's Move

www.let'smove.gov

MYPlate (USDA)

www.choosemyplate.gov/kids

Yale Rudd Center for Food Policy and Obesity

www.yaleruddcenter.org

About the Author

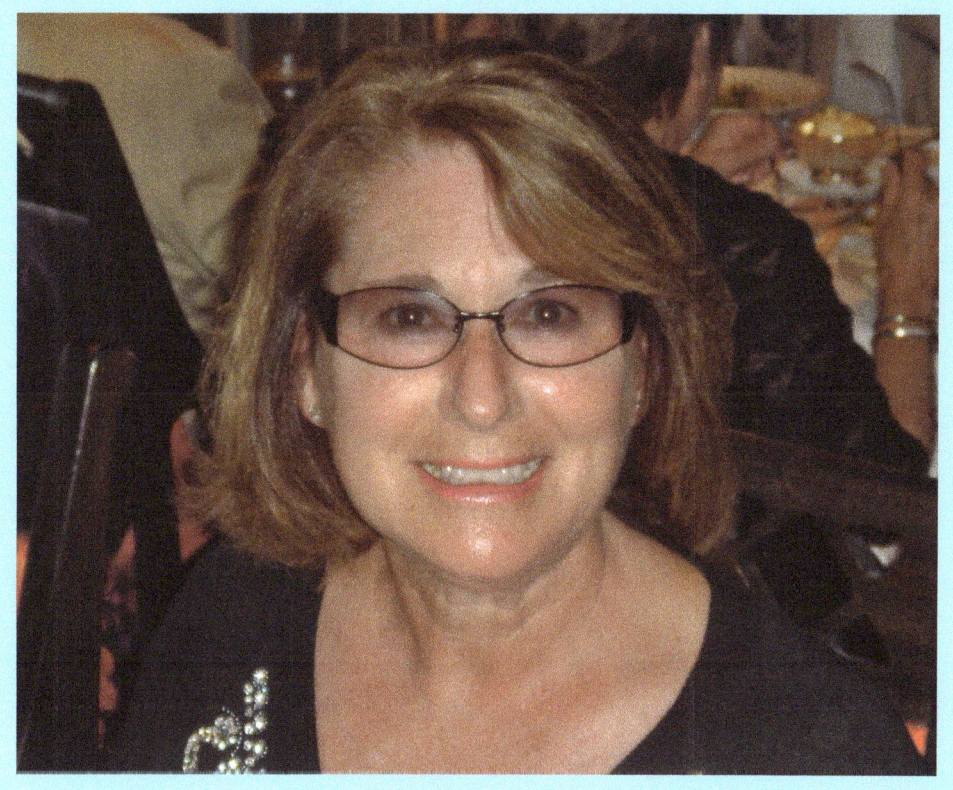

As an advanced-level nutrition practitioner, **Dr. Roni Roth Beshears** has worked at the local, state, and federal levels with food and nutrition programs and services. As a community volunteer and advocate, she has devoted time and energy to serving the needs of vulnerable women, children and families. Dr. Roth Beshears is a registered dietitian nutritionist and certified health and wellness coach. She is a graduate of Syracuse University (BS) and Columbia University, Teachers College (EdD).

www.ingramcontent.com/pod-product-compliance
Lightning Source LLC
Chambersburg PA
CBHW061400160426
42811CB00099B/1293

Anabelle Takes a Hike

By Mitzi Cherry Moye
Illustrations by Lauren Adair Jones
Edited by Melissa Howard Lambert

Copyright © 2014 Mitzi Moye
All rights reserved.
ISBN: 978-0-9864490-0-0 Cherry Publishing

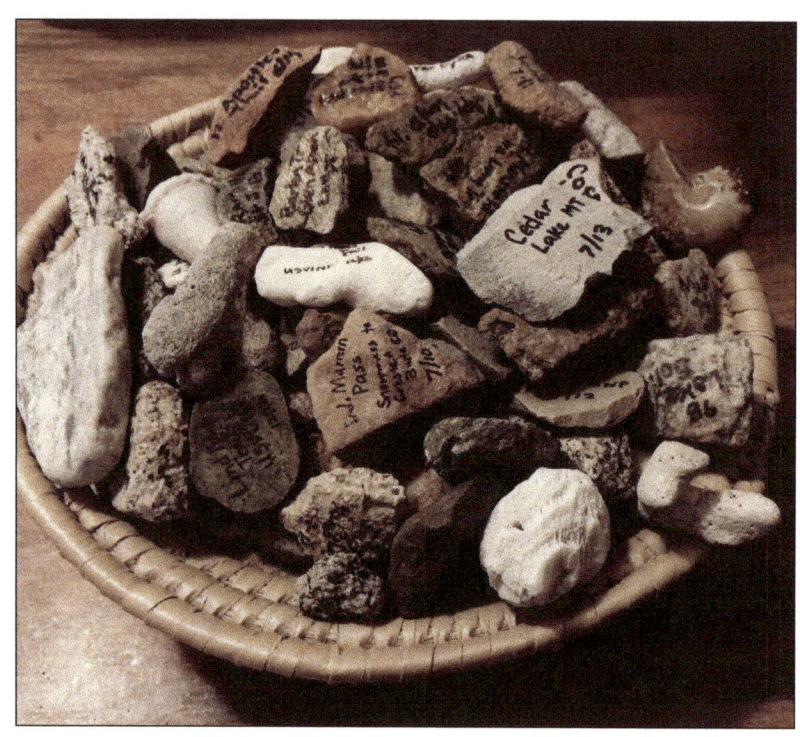

DEDICATION

This book is in honor of the many brave women I have known- my mother, Lena Davis Cherry who lived a long life filled with heroic deeds, daughter Holly who bravely fights for lives every day, and daughter Brittany who shares in that battle.

Melissa's editing expertise and Lauren's creativity made this book possible.

There is a huge cast of supporting characters in this league of women – Pam, Mattie, Beth C, Gibbs, and Mama Jo, Georgia and Elizabeth, Ann W, Beth M and Lisa T, Cindy, Lisa B, Michelle, Vicki, Karen, Leslie and Melissa, and most dearly - my brave and beloved fellow hikers: Carolyn, Nina, Jaclynn and Winston.

You mean the world to me.

ACKNOWLEDGMENTS

Everyone knows it – he's the love of my life... To Andy

To my grandchildren, great nieces and nephews -
May you be brave, appreciate art, and enjoy this beautiful world

Anabelle is a brave girl.

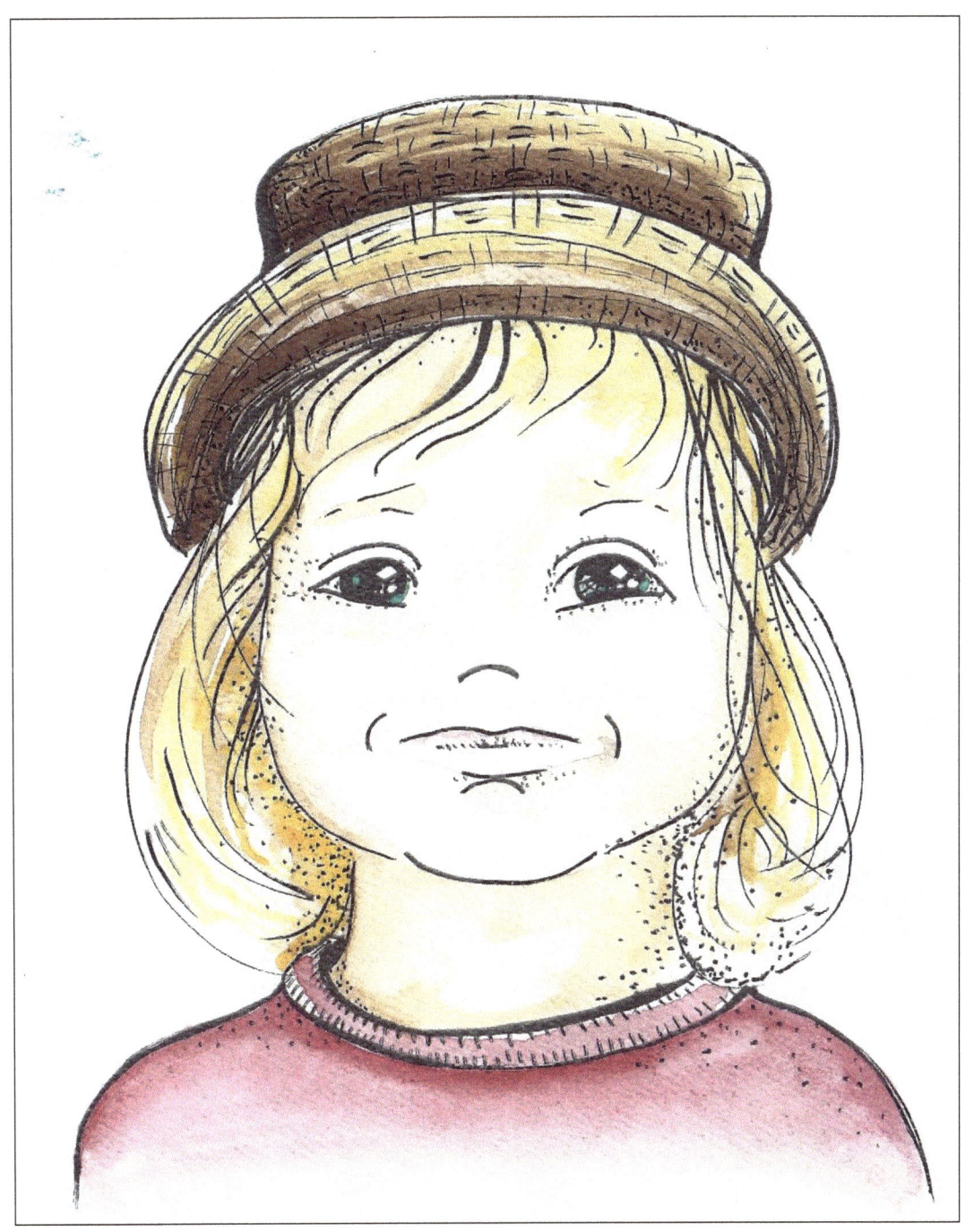

Sometimes she feels a little scared of something, like a creepy bug, or a dark shadow, or a loud noise.

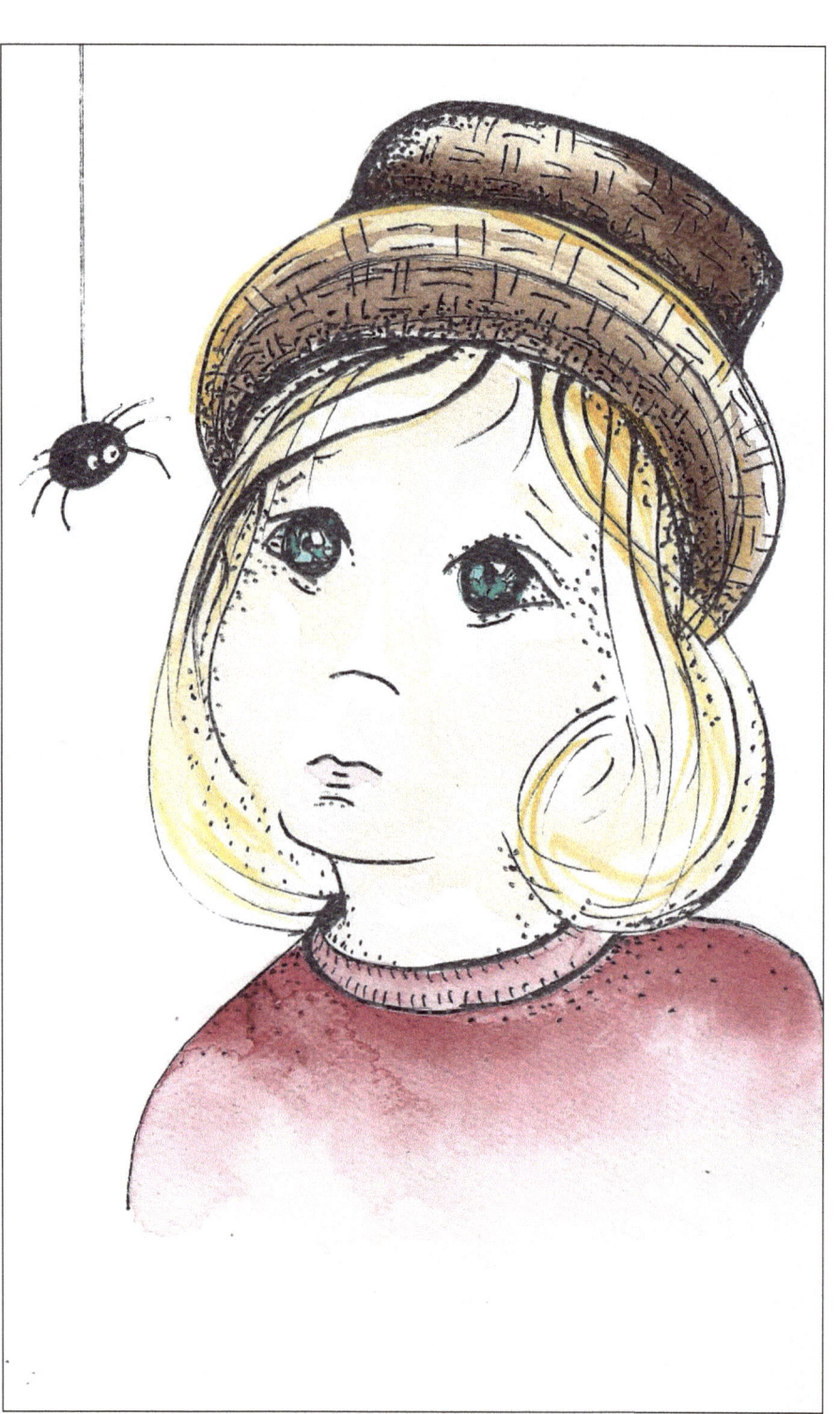

But mostly, she is brave.

She does brave things,

like taste broccoli,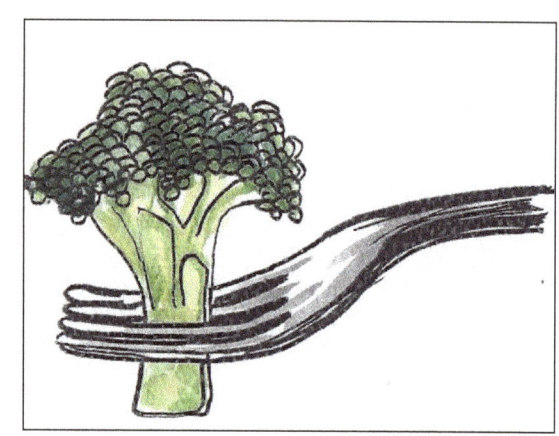

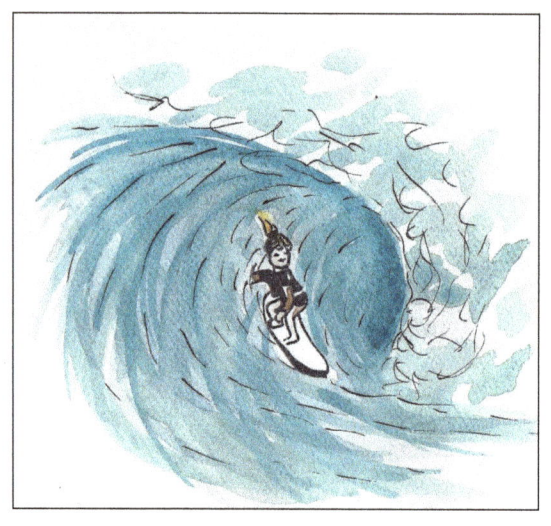 or surf a wave,

or meet a new friend.

Sometimes Anabelle helps others who aren't so brave. She helped Lila take her first bite of watermelon.

Anabelle likes watermelon.

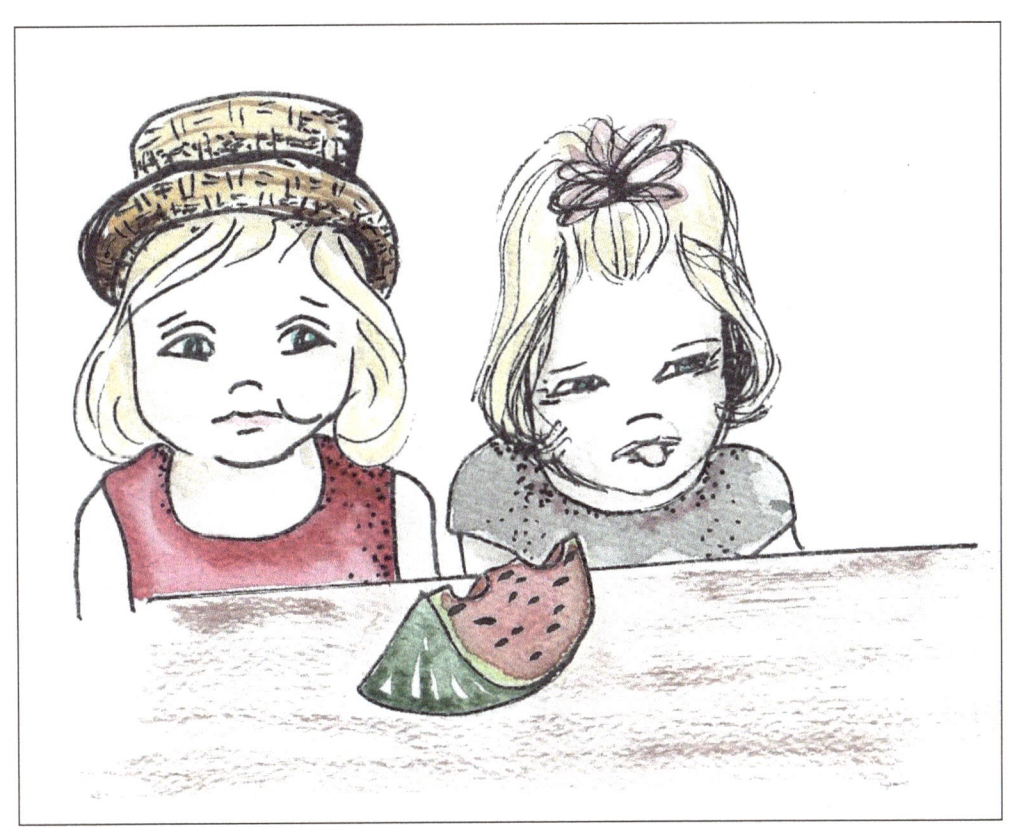

Lila didn't like it.

Anabelle helps Lawson enjoy the beach. The first time he jumped a wave, he was a little bit scared.

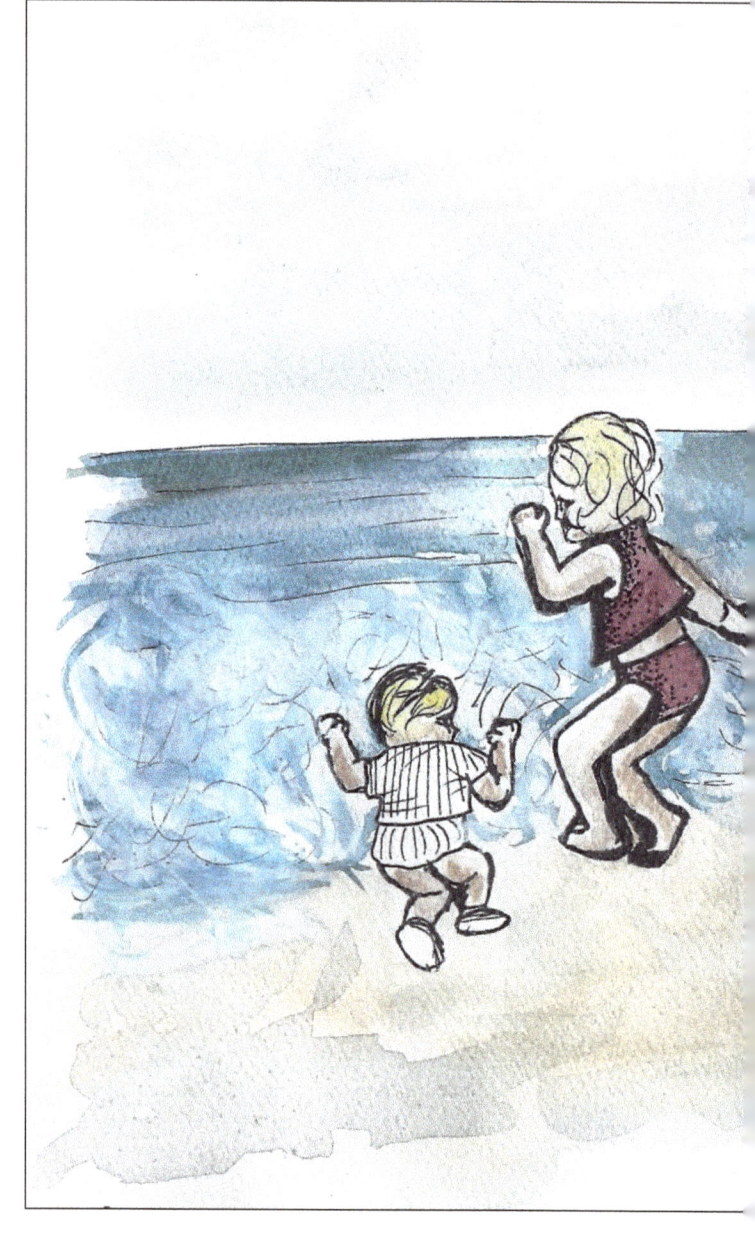

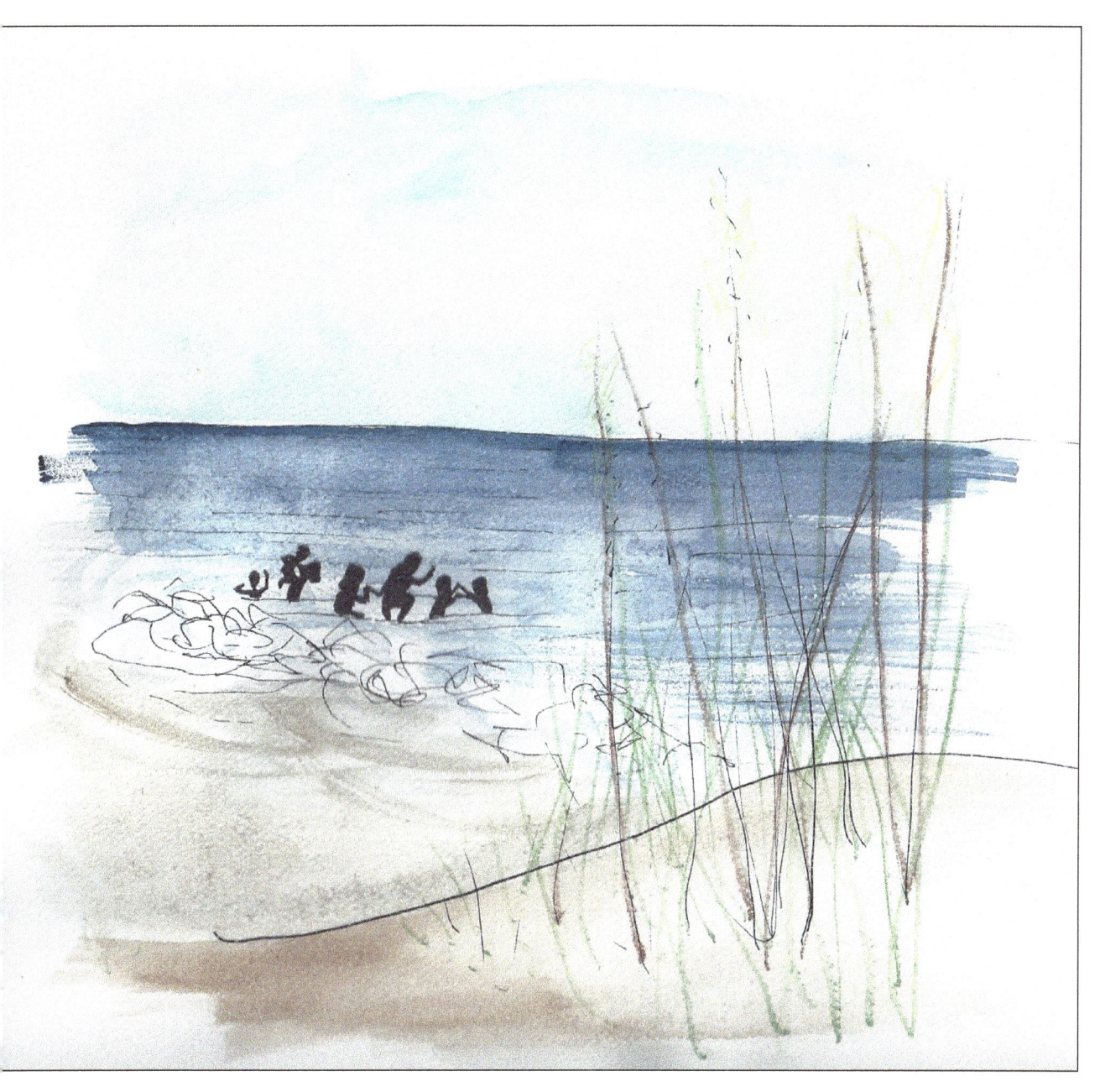

But by the fourth time, he loved it.

Anabelle tries to play golf with her bigger cousin Will.

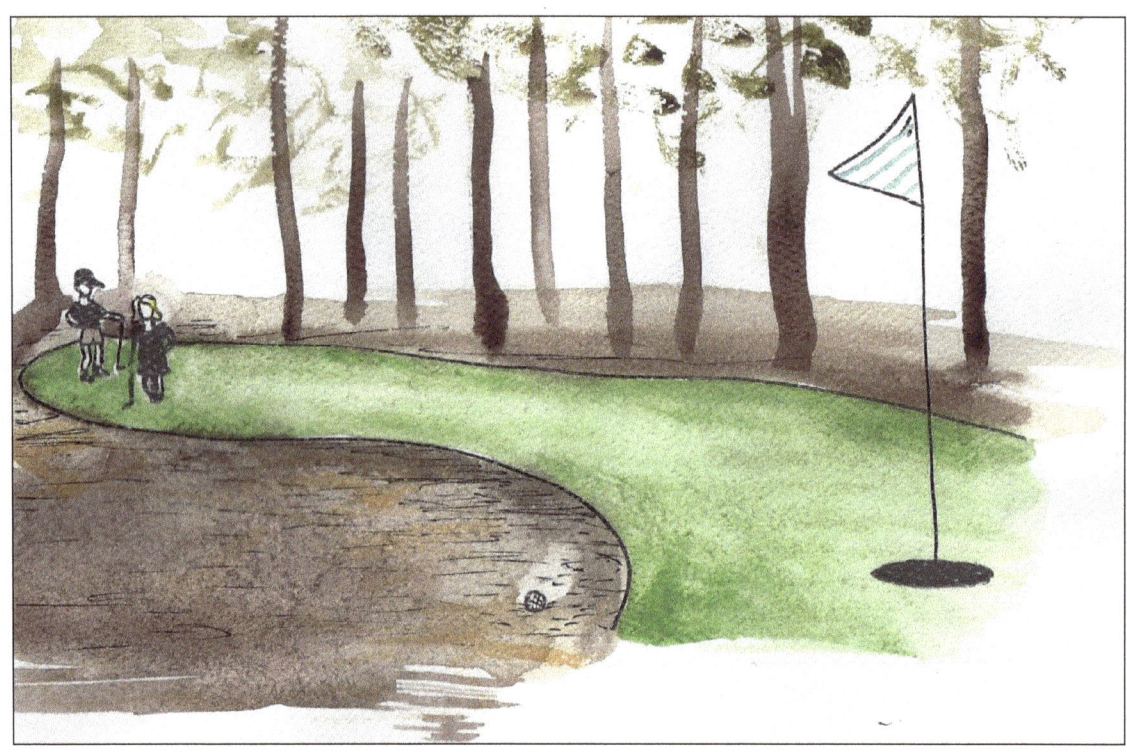

She isn't very good, but at least she tries.

Anabelle doesn't like everything she tries. She doesn't like high heels or pink medicine. She doesn't like sitting still and listening for a long, long time.

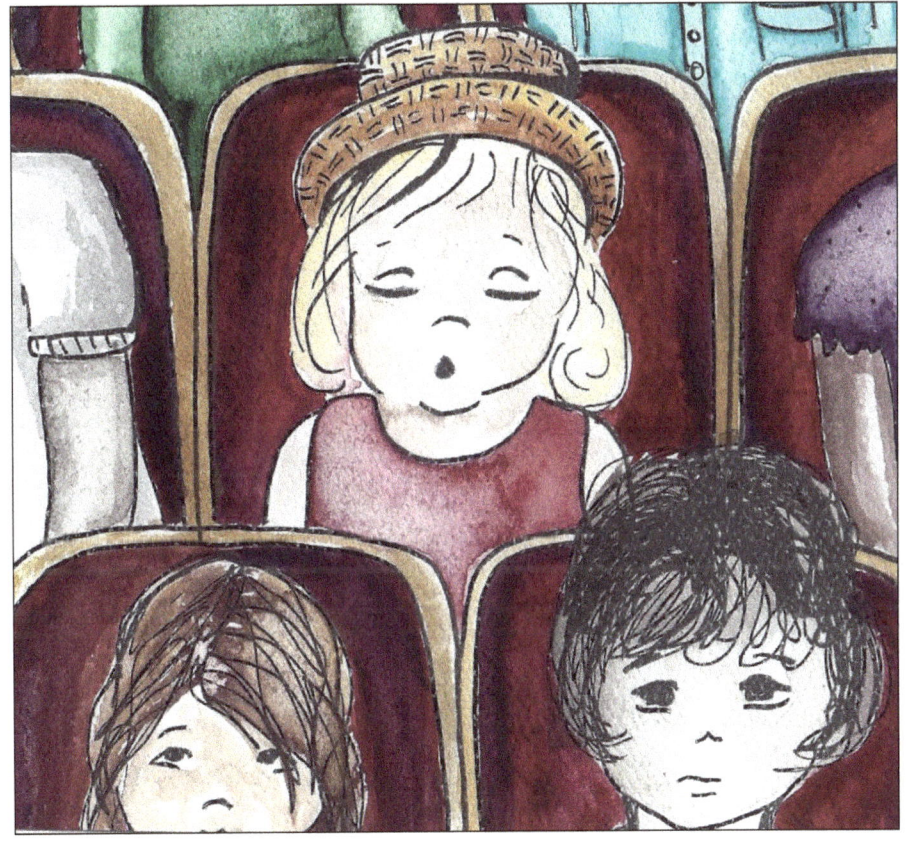

But she keeps trying. As she tries more things, her bravery grows.

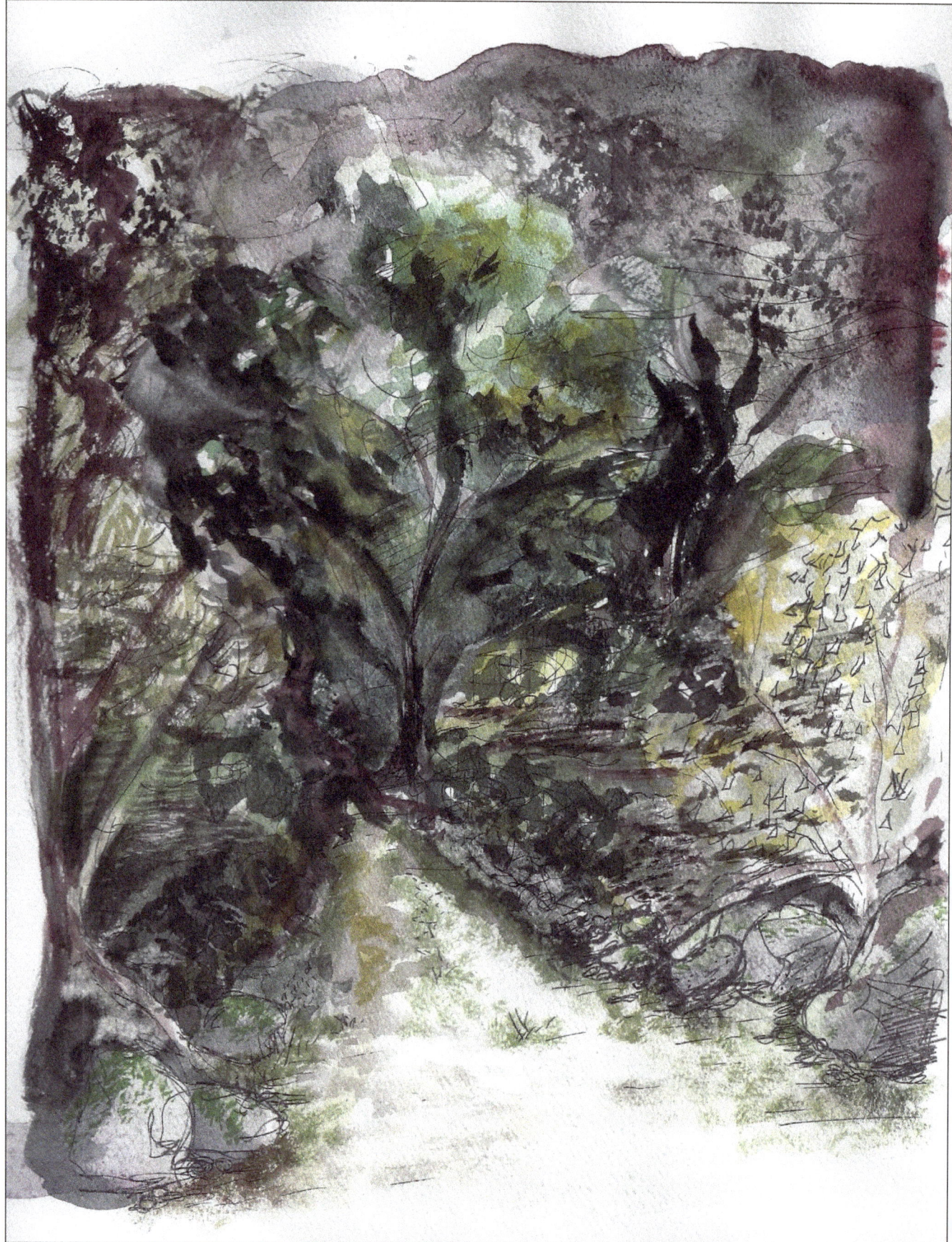

There are woods near Anabelle's house, with a trail going into the trees. One day, she was feeling especially brave, and decided to go for a hike.

The trees were huge and the path was rocky, but she wanted to explore this new place.

Anabelle wanted to try.

It looked a little scary.

She invited her cousins to come along because...

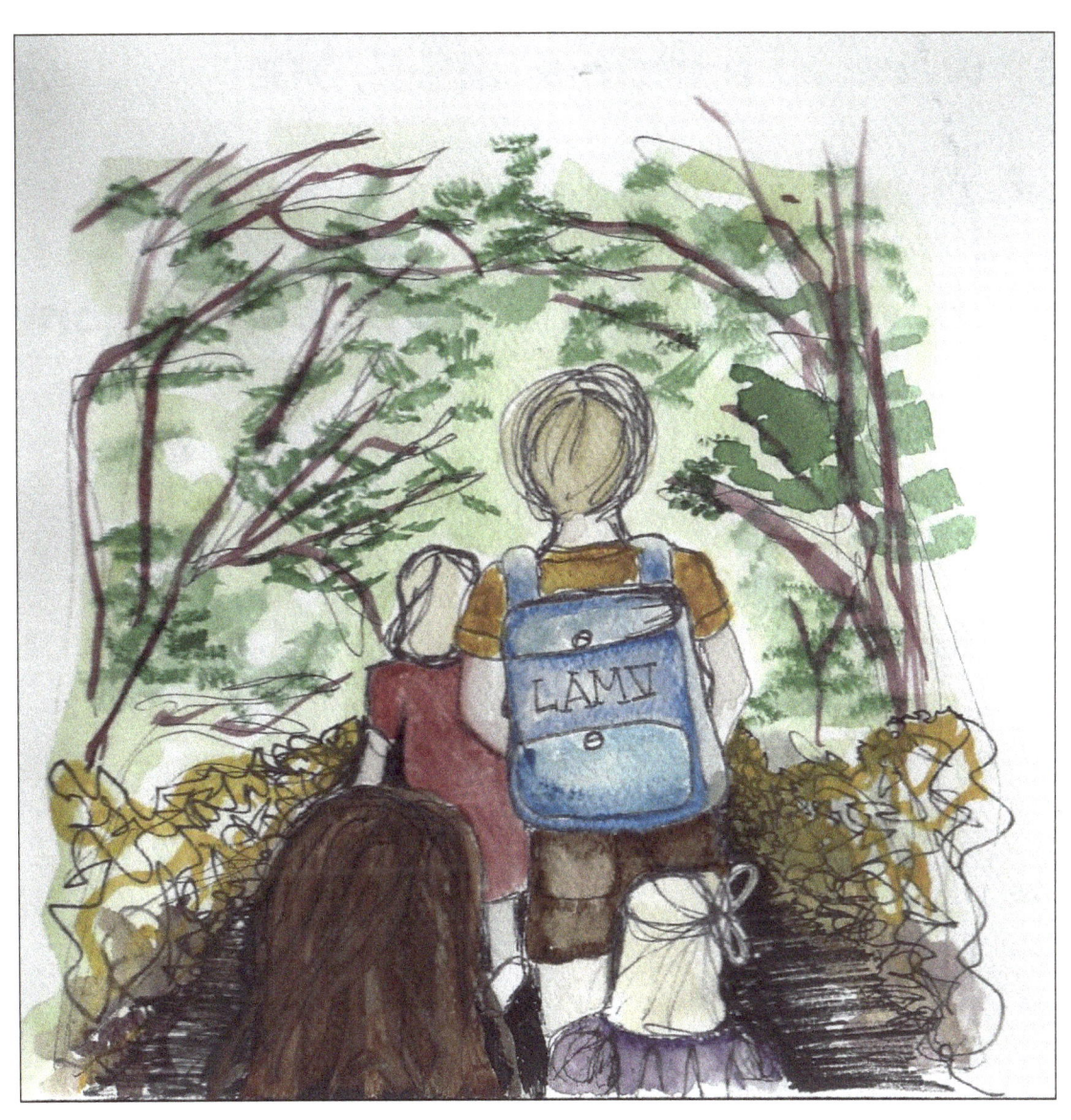

sometimes things are a little less scary if you have your family or friends with you.

They were all a little scared, but Anabelle promised to lead them (and they asked Grandma to come along).

Together, they planned for what they would need on the hike. They packed water and 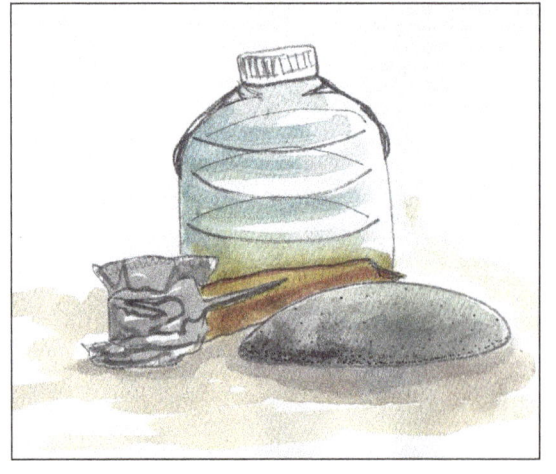 snacks in their backpacks and made sure that their shoes were tied tight.

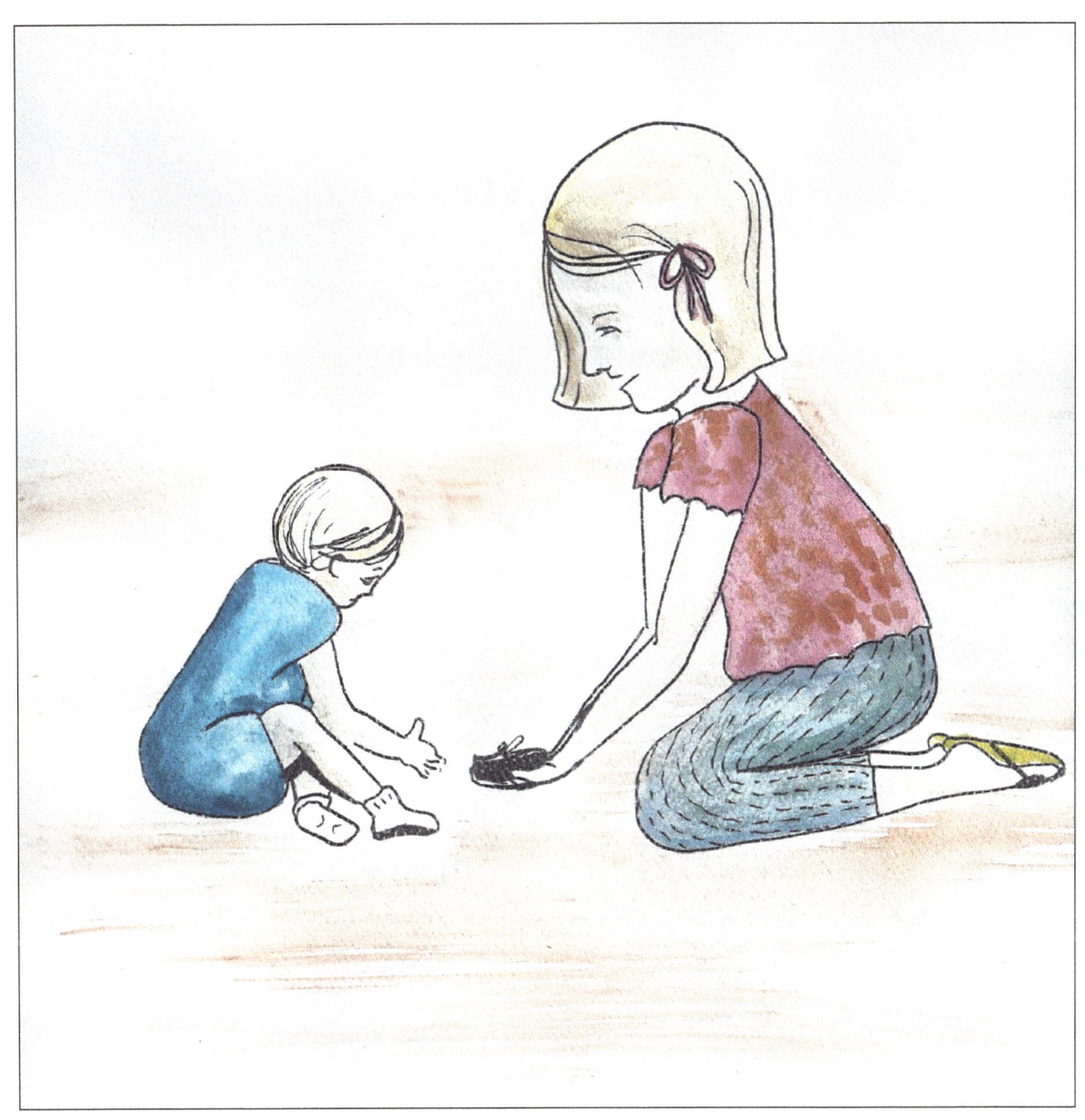

Lawson was the youngest and did not know how to tie his shoes.

Charlotte helped him.

Off they went into the woods. The trees were so tall. They had to step over big roots and pay attention to the trail.

It was an adventure!

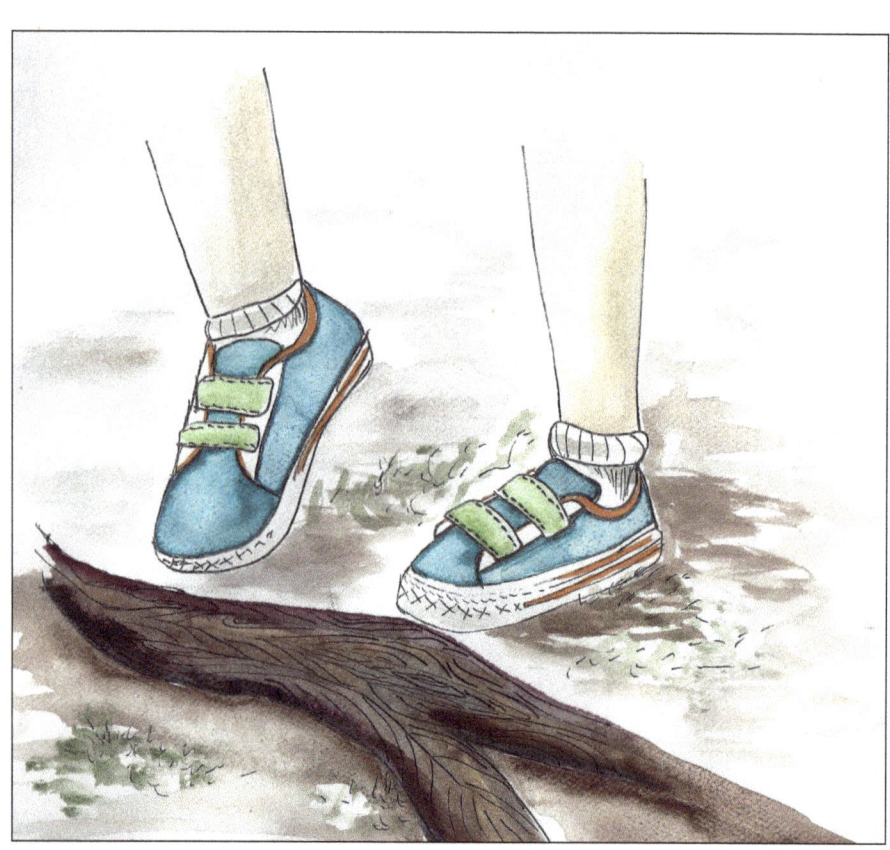

While they walked they sang songs and laughed. Their legs were tired, but being together made it fun. Anabelle was not even afraid of the bugs. She felt safe with her cousins.

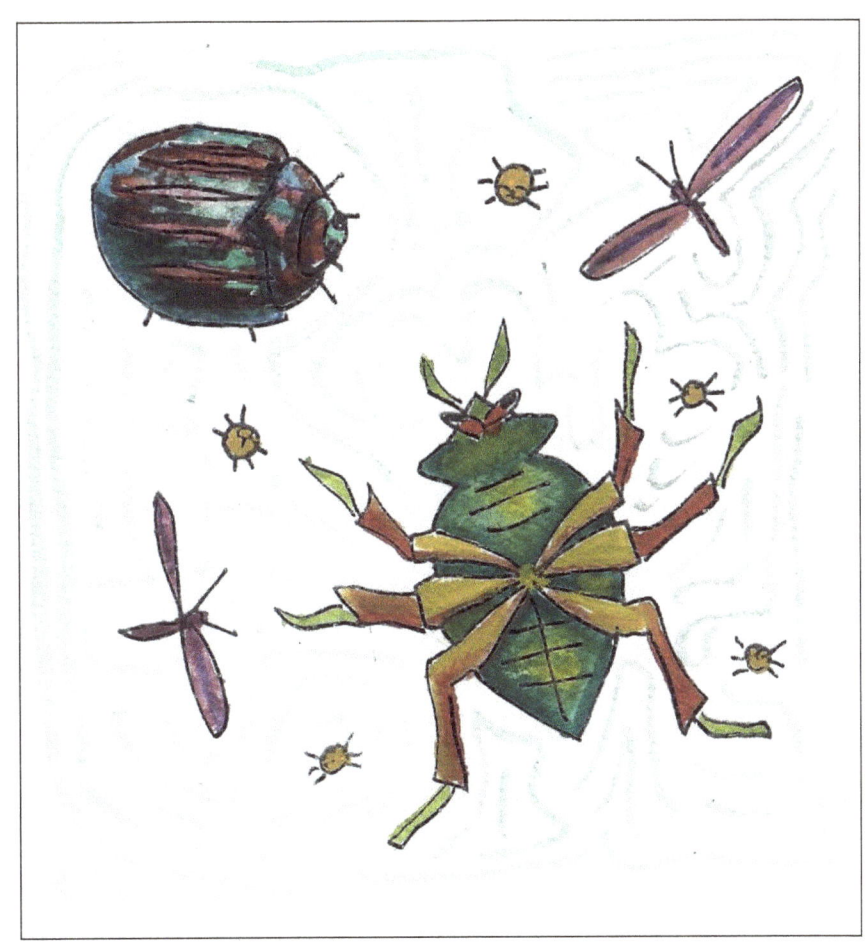

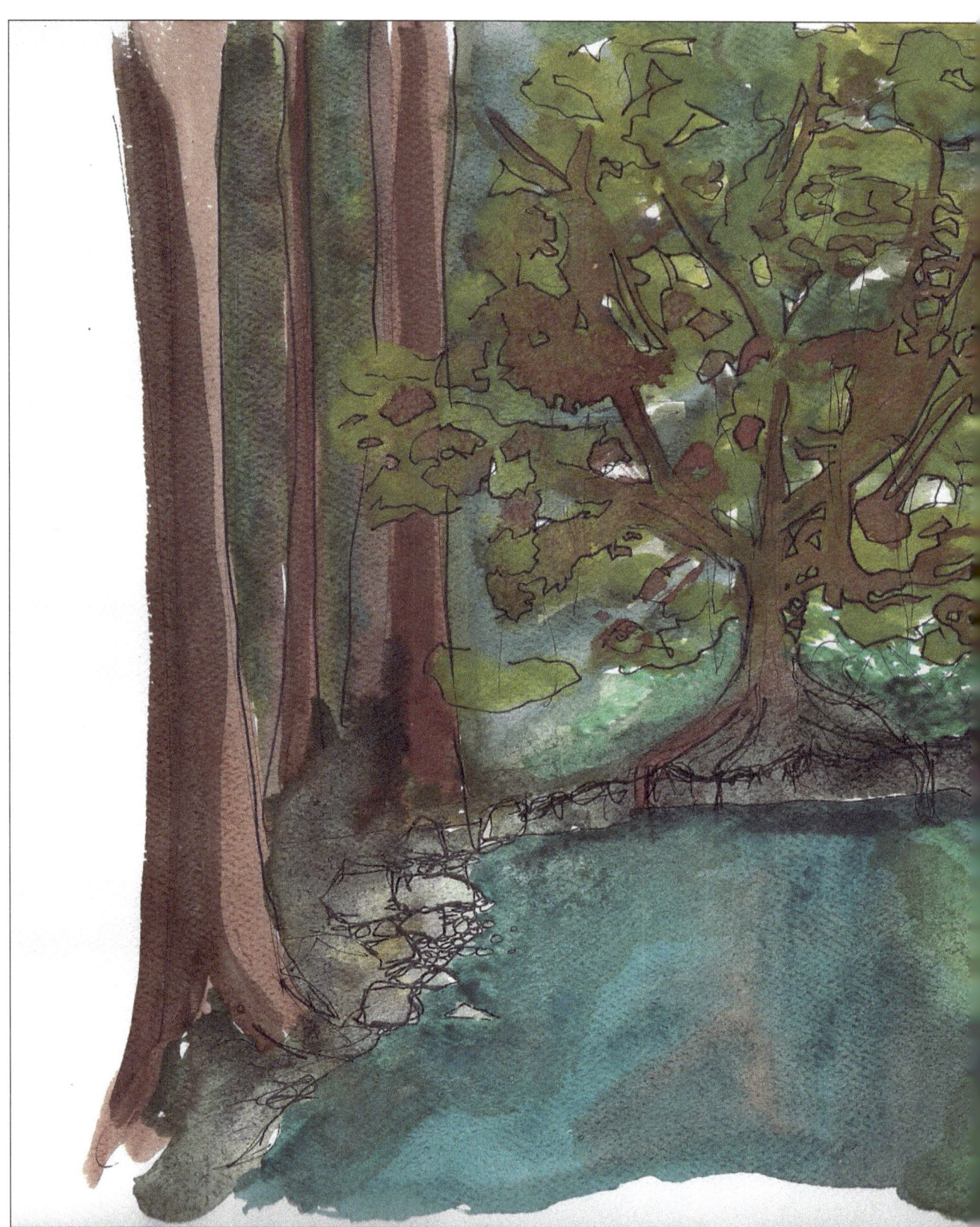

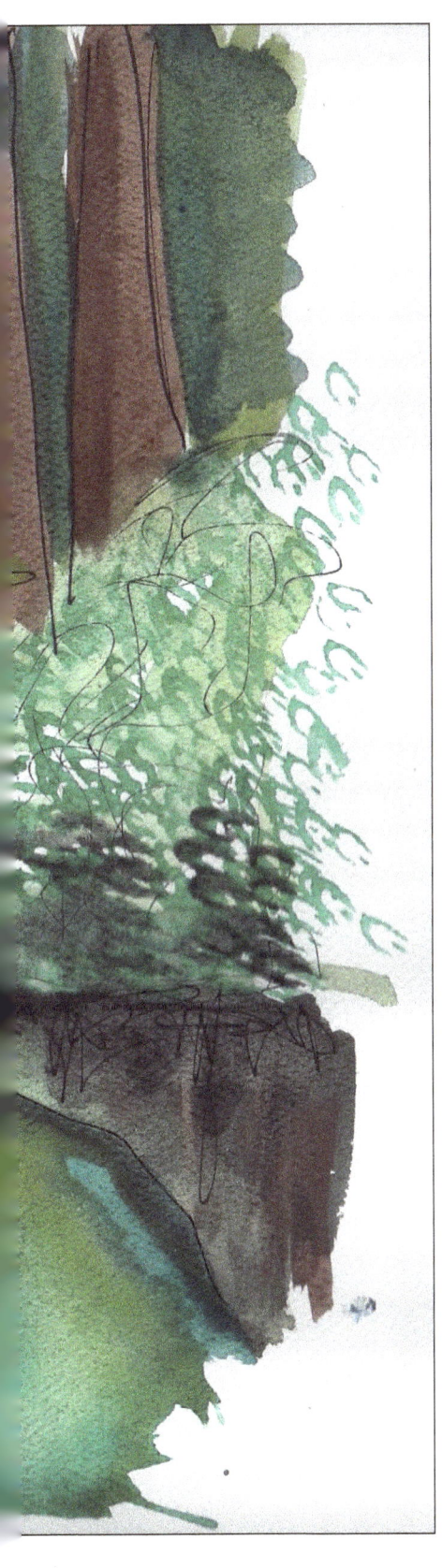

They reached a clearing in the woods and discovered a pond. "I never knew this was here," said Anabelle. The cousins cheered, "We found a special place!"

They sat beside the pond and shared snacks. All around them were new things – birds singing, frogs croaking and even a fish jumping out of the water.

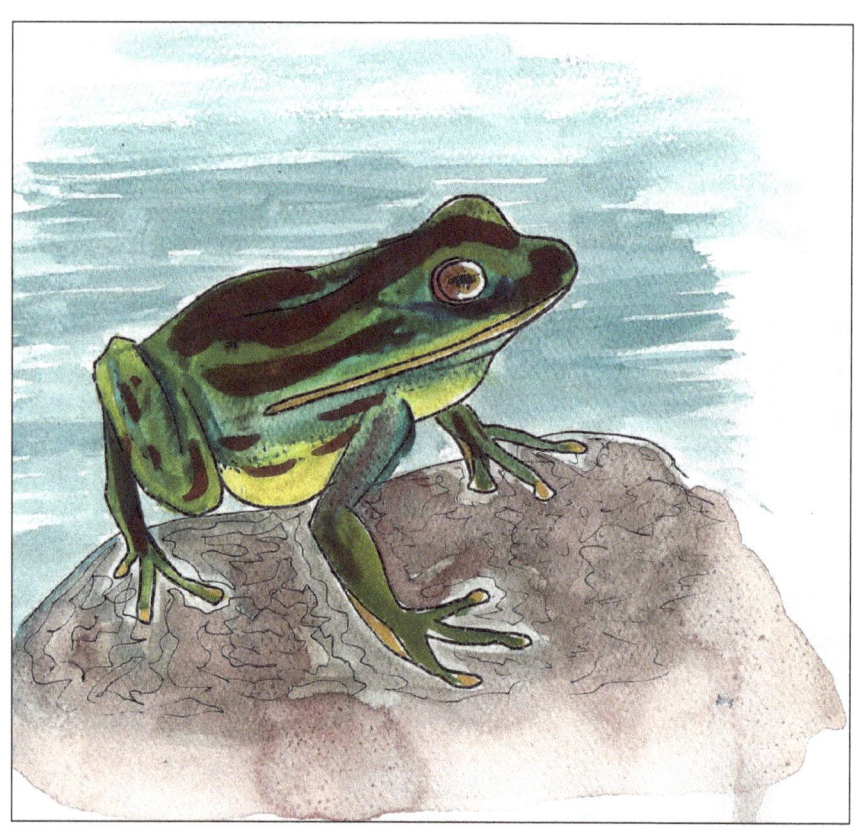

It wasn't scary at all!

"We need to be sure that we are back before dark," said Anabelle.

Before they left, they cleaned up from their snack, and each found one smooth rock to take as a reminder of the hiking adventure.

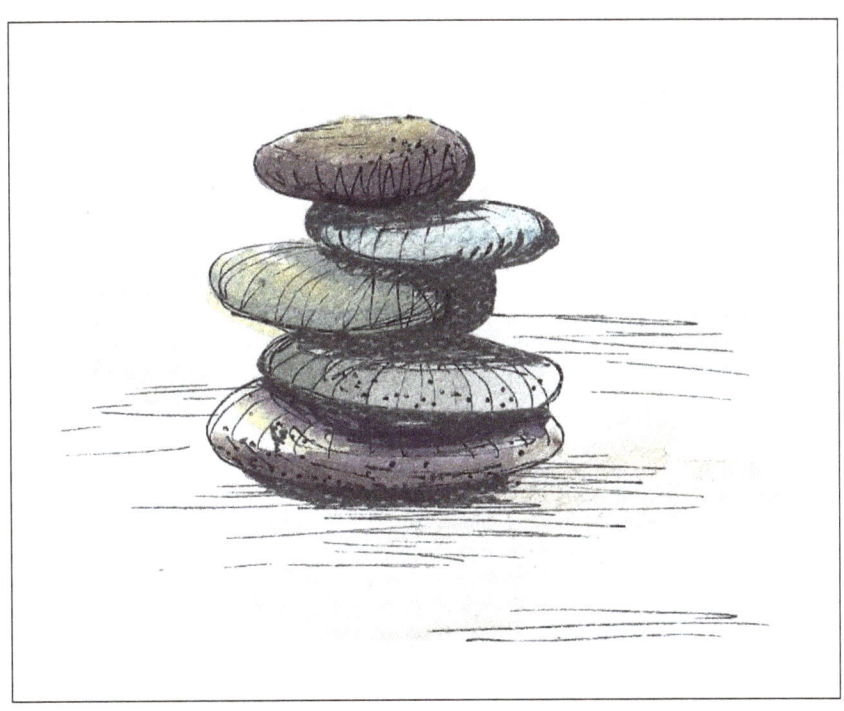

As the cousins grew up, their rocks reminded them of their bravery.

Sara put her rock in her backpack for her first day of school.

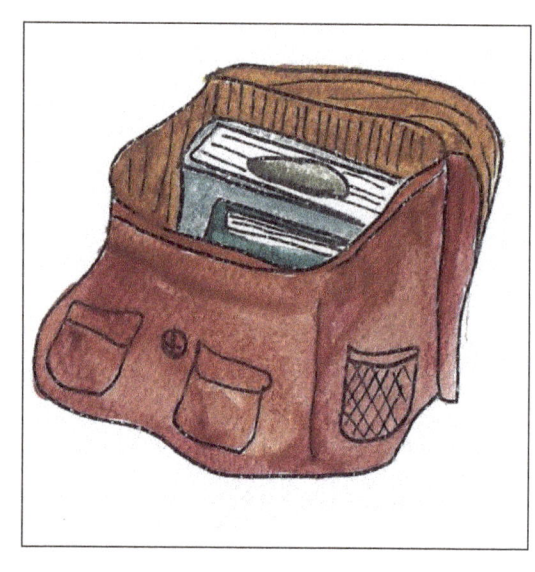

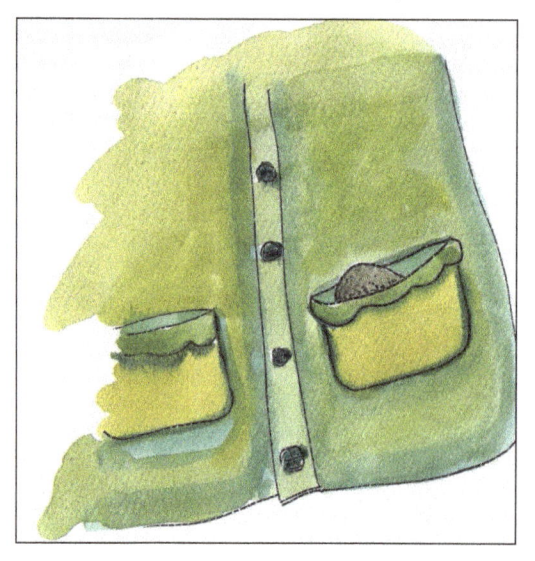

Davis put his rock in his pocket when he made his first trip to the dentist.

Lawson collected more and more rocks.

He loved exploring new places.

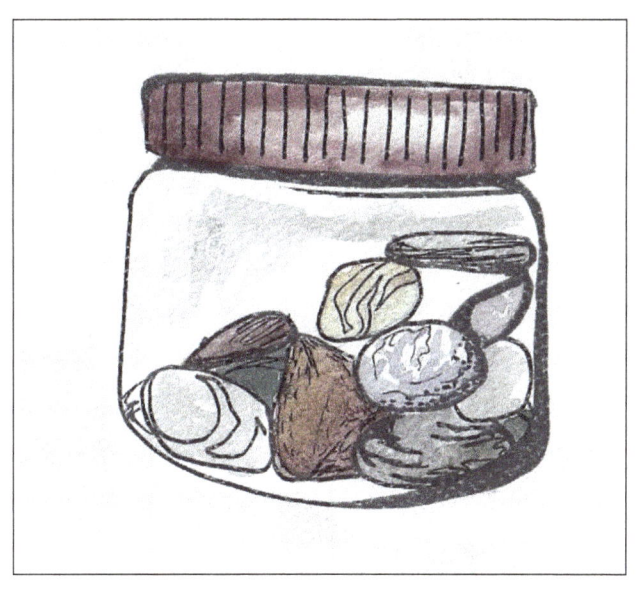

For every new adventure, the rocks reminded each of them of a time when something was a bit scary, but they were brave.

Almost every day, they tried something new. They were glad that Anabelle was brave and hiked with them. And as they slept each night, they dreamed of the exciting adventures ahead.

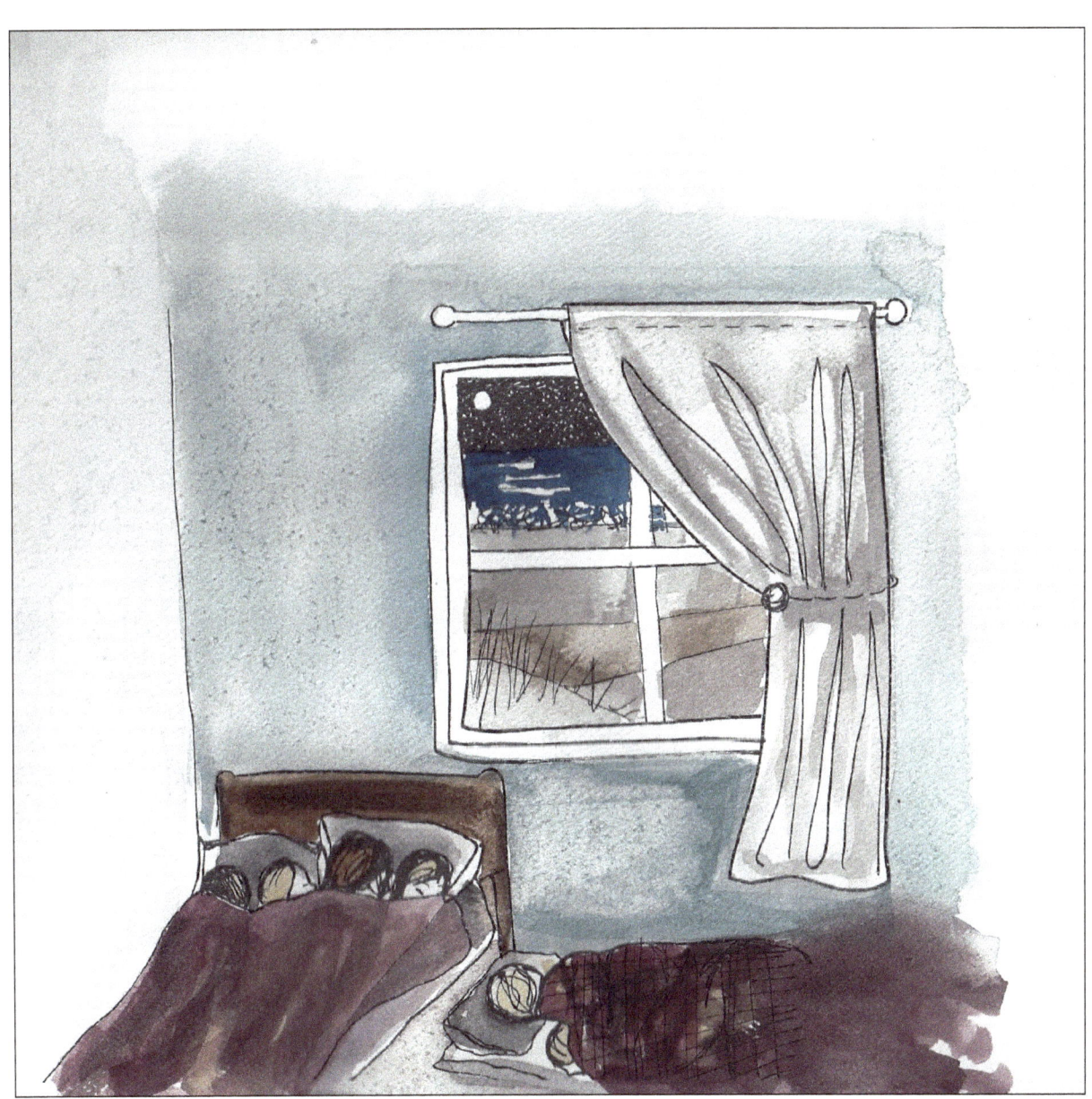

www.ingramcontent.com/pod-product-compliance
Lightning Source LLC
Chambersburg PA
CBHW061400160426
42811CB00099B/1295

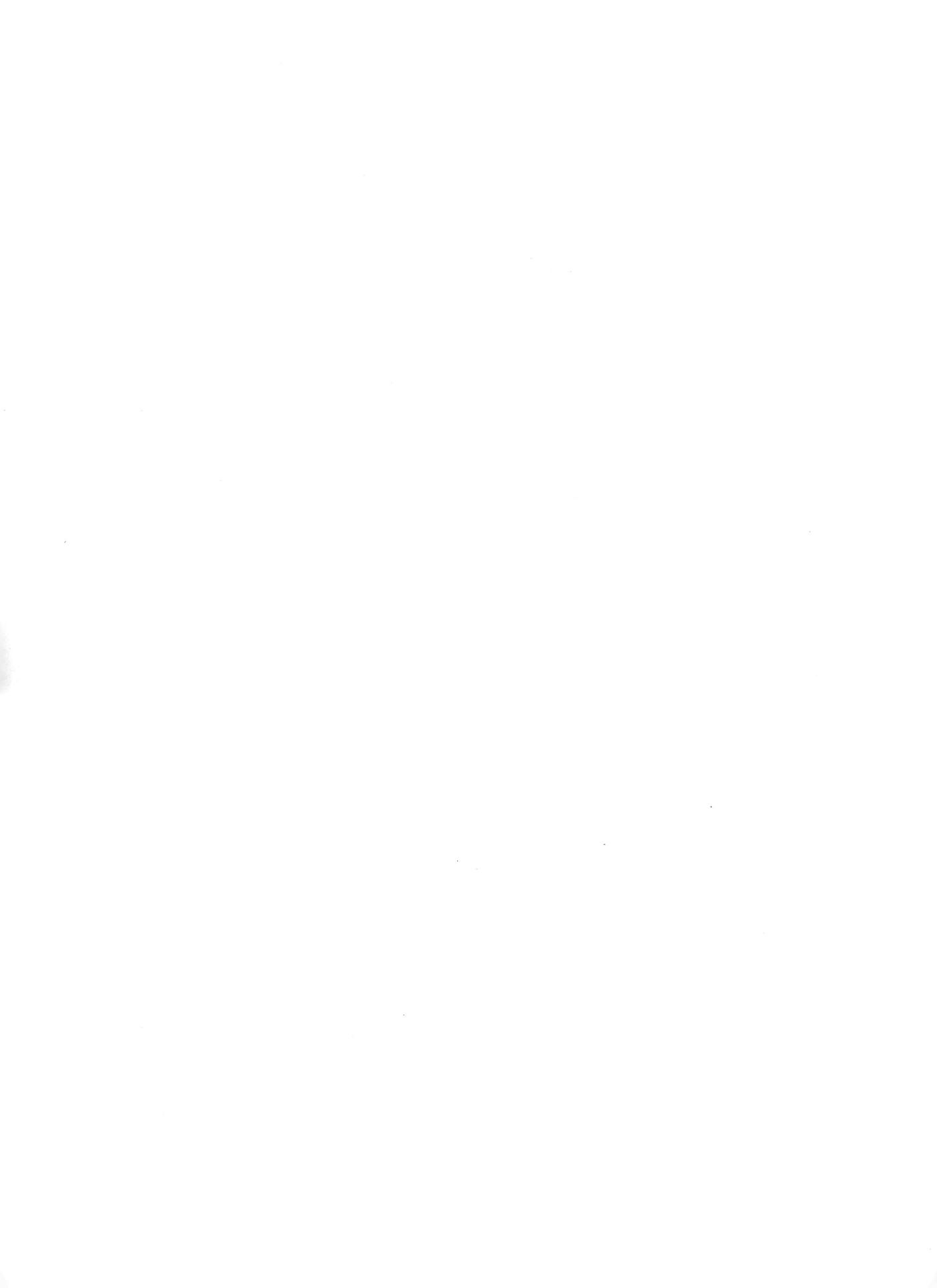